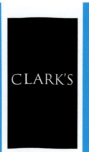

ESSENTIAL
PHYSICS IN
IMAGING FOR

CLARK'S

RADIOGRAPHERS

Clark's Essential Guides

PUBLISHED

Clark's Essential Physics in Imaging for Radiographers (2013)
Ken Holmes, *School of Medical Imaging Sciences,*
University of Cumbria, Lancaster, UK

Marcus Elkington, *Medical Imaging Department,*
Sheffield Hallam University, Sheffield, UK

Phil Harris, *Health & Medical Sciences, Quality Group,*
University of Cumbria, Lancaster, UK

Clark's Pocket Handbook for Radiographers (2010)
Charles Sloane, Stewart A Whitley, Craig Anderson, and Ken Holmes,
School of Medical Imaging Sciences, University of Cumbria, Lancaster, UK

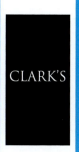

CLARK'S ESSENTIAL PHYSICS IN IMAGING FOR RADIOGRAPHERS

Ken Holmes
University of Cumbria, UK

Marcus Elkington
Sheffield Hallam University, UK

Phil Harris
University of Cumbria, UK

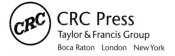

CRC Press
Taylor & Francis Group
Boca Raton London New York

CRC Press is an imprint of the
Taylor & Francis Group, an **informa** business

CRC Press
Taylor & Francis Group
6000 Broken Sound Parkway NW, Suite 300
Boca Raton, FL 33487-2742

© 2014 by Ken Holmes, Marcus Elkington, and Phil Harris
CRC Press is an imprint of Taylor & Francis Group, an Informa business

No claim to original U.S. Government works

Printed on acid-free paper
Version Date: 20130401

Printed and bound in India by Replika Press Pvt. Ltd.

International Standard Book Number-13: 978-1-4441-4561-8 (Paperback)

Library of Congress Cataloging-in-Publication Data

Holmes, Ken (Kenneth), 1955-
Clark's essential physics in imaging for radiographers / Ken Holmes, Marcus Elkington, Phil Harris.
p. ; cm.
Essential physics in imaging for radiographers
Includes bibliographical references and index.
ISBN 978-1-4441-4561-8 (pbk. : alk. paper)
I. Clark, Kathleen C. (Kathleen Clara) II. Elkington, Marcus. III. Harris, Phil, 1955- IV. Title. V. Title: Essential physics in imaging for radiographers.
[DNLM: 1. Radiography--Handbooks. 2. Radiation--Handbooks. WN 39]

RC78.A1
616.07'572--dc23   2013011207

Visit the Taylor & Francis Web site at
http://www.taylorandfrancis.com

and the CRC Press Web site at
http://www.crcpress.com

CONTENTS

PREFACE

The authors all have several years' experience teaching undergraduate physics and have seen the evolution from film to digital imaging. Although there are some relevant books available, the information often requires careful filtering by the student. We have tried to write a book where the topics are covered in 'bite' size chunks. The idea is to provide a clear guide to the subject using clear text and diagrams/photographs to support the text. Each chapter has clear 'learning objectives' and a series of multiple choice questions (MCQs) to test these learning outcomes.

The aim of this book is to give the reader an understanding of the basic physics underpinning diagnostic radiography and imaging science. It is essential that any practitioner working in an imaging department and using ionising radiation has a sound knowledge base. In order to understand the various factors affecting the production of diagnostic images, there is a requirement to demonstrate an understanding of the fundamental definitions of physics and how these principles may be applied to radiography.

The book opens with chapters that give an overview of image production, basic mathematics and physics relevant to medical imaging and then detailed chapters on the physics relevant to producing diagnostic images using X-rays. Diagnostic radiography involves the safe use of ionising radiation and the production of diagnostic images. The process by which images are produced involves the conversion of energy from one form to another and this underpins the fundamentals of imaging. It requires knowledge of specialised equipment, such as the X-ray tube, image detectors, computers and image processors. Understanding the fundamental principles of this equipment is the basic knowledge base of any practitioner.

The final chapters review the factors affecting image quality and radiation dose: how correct exposures are indicated by the equipment together with how to manipulate images, data management and display parameters. Discussion of risk benefit, safety and radiation protection conclude the book as these are necessary requirements of health-care practitioners using ionising radiation.

THE AUTHORS

Ken Holmes is the programme leader for the BSc (Hons) Diagnostic Imaging at the University of Cumbria (formerly St Martins College). He is one of the co-authors of *Clark's Pocket Handbook for Radiographers* and believes the time is right to develop a pocket physics book to use alongside the technique one. Ken started education as a clinical tutor and has worked at several higher education institutes in the UK and has taught physics and imaging principles for 30 years. He still works clinically with students and enjoys the challenge of explaining imaging technology and physics to them.

Marcus Elkington is a senior lecturer in Diagnostic Imaging at Sheffield Hallam University. He has a great interest in imaging and physics related to diagnostic radiography and has been helping students understand physics for many years. Marcus feels there is a place for a pocket physics book produced in a student-friendly format that is aimed specifically at the core topic areas surrounding general radiographic imaging.

Phil Harris has been a senior lecturer and head of school at Medical Imaging Science at the University of Cumbria for many years and has always taken the greatest pleasure in passing on a basic understanding of radiation science to radiography students, many of whom enter into this subject with some considerable trepidation. This book has been written especially with these students in mind.

CHAPTER 1
OVERVIEW OF IMAGE PRODUCTION

INTRODUCTION

The aim of this chapter is to give the practitioner an understanding of the basic principles of image production. It is essential that any practitioner understands the principles involved in obtaining diagnostic images. Images must be produced using the lowest radiation dose consistent with diagnostic quality. The practitioner therefore needs to understand how to adjust the factors affecting dose and image quality.

> **Learning objectives**
>
> The student should be able to:
> - Understand and explain the principles of producing images using X-radiation.
> - Explain the terms magnification, unsharpness, scatter, contrast, definition and resolution.

GENERAL PRINCIPLES

The objective of diagnostic imaging is to produce images of optimum quality for diagnosis and to aid in the management/treatment of the patient. There must be a valid reason for the examination. The procedure must also affect the clinical management of the patient. The procedure should produce images with limited magnification, minimum unsharpness and a radiation dose as low as reasonably practicable (ALARP).

The ideal set-up is to have the body part being imaged parallel to and in contact with the image detector. The X-ray beam should be at right angles to the detector and not angled across it as this produces a distorted image. However, there are situations where the patient or X-ray beam is angled to deliberately distort/elongate the image, e.g. 30° angled elongated scaphoid projection.

There are a number of factors which affect the quality of the image and/or radiation dose to the patient when producing diagnostic images using X-rays. These are:

- The X-ray beam characteristics:
    - Focal spot size
    - Filtration of the beam
    - Exposure factors
    - Field size
    - The production and management/reduction of scatter
    - The geometry of image production.
- The patient:
    - Ability to keep still
    - Thickness and density of the body parts
- The detector and imaging system:
    - Using computed radiography (CR) and digital radiography (DR) technology
    - Quantum Detection Efficiency (QDE)
    - The display system
    - Viewing conditions
- The practitioner's skill and perception.

X-RAY BEAM CHARACTERISTICS

The production of X-rays will be described in a later chapter however, in terms of image production there are a number of requirements of the X-ray beam.

- The beam needs to be filtered to preferentially remove low energy photons which will not penetrate the patient. This reduces radiation dose and changes the energy range of the X-rays in the beam, which hardens the beam (makes the beam more homogenous, i.e. there are a smaller range of intensities).

- The source of radiation (focus) from the X-ray tube is small (typically from 0.3 mm^2 fine focus to 2 mm^2 broad focus).
- The size of the radiation beam can be collimated to the body part to reduce scatter and intensity.
- The energy of the beam needs to be adjustable to enable a range of exposures:
  - Kilovoltage from 40 to 125
  - Milliamperage from 50 to 1000
  - Exposure times from 0.001 to several seconds.

SCATTERED RADIATION

The primary beam of radiation leaving the X-ray tube interacts with the patient. There are only three possibilities for the X-ray photons leaving the X-ray tube:

1. The photons are absorbed by the patient and cease to exist (this may cause radiation damage). This gives information about the density and thickness of the patient and help create an image (signal).
2. The photons pass through the patient and produce a point of information in the detector and also help create an image (signal).
3. The photons are scattered within the patient or detector.
   a. This contributes to noise if they interact with the detector.
   b. Absorbed photons in the patient again may cause radiation damage with no benefit to the image.

The image on the detector can therefore been seen as an attenuation 'map' of radiation which has passed through the patient.

FIELD SIZE

The area of the patient irradiated can be controlled by collimation of the X-ray beam. The maximum field size at 100 cm focus receptor distance (FRD) is 43 cm^2. However, it is critical that the beam of radiation is limited only to the area of interest. This can improve image quality and reduce the radiation dose to the patient and therefore staff by minimising the amount of scattered radiation produced.

GEOMETRY OF IMAGE PRODUCTION

All radiographic images produced using an X-ray source and detector will be larger than the object being imaged. However, this is not always apparent from the image on the monitor as the image is optimised for image viewing by the computing system and may appear 'life-size'. There are some important aspects determined by the geometry of the imaging system which are relevant when producing the image.

- Magnification
- Unsharpness
- Resolution/definition.

All of these factors are altered when selecting the equipment and factors for the set up of the X-ray examination. **Table 1.1** states terms related to geometry.

Magnification

As stated above, all images produced are larger than the body part being X-rayed. One key skill of the practitioner is to produce images with minimal magnification and unsharpness. Any unsharpness produced is magnified by the object receptor distance.

Magnification is reduced by close contact between the patient's body part and the image receptor. In practice, a standardised FRD should be used. A FRD of 100 cm for table work and 180 cm for erect chest images is used (**Figure 1.1**). Distances must be standardised within departments to standardise magnification.

The magnification in an image may be represented by the formula:

$$Magnification = \frac{FRD}{FOD} \cdot$$

Table 1.1 Terms related to geometry. (See Figure 1.1)

Distances	Abbreviation
Focus to receptor distance	FRD
Focus to object distance	FOD
Object to receptor distance	ORD

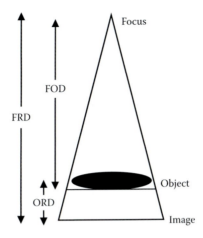

Figure 1.1 Distances used in radiographic image production.

Unsharpness

All images produced in radiography have a level of unsharpness, which should not be visible to the practitioner. This is approximately 0.3 mm and is determined by a number of factors:

- Movement of the patient
  - The patient may need to be immobilised or asked to arrest respiration to avoid movement unsharpness.
- Geometry of imaging
  - Related to distances of the patient, focus and detector
- How the data are displayed
  - Type of monitor and its characteristics
- Brightness and contrast of the monitor
- Viewing conditions
  - Background conditions, e.g. light intensity in the room
  - Resolution and quality of the monitor
- Perception of the practitioner
  - Affected by the contrast, resolution of the image and their experience of viewing images.

The unsharpness (penumbra) of the image can be calculated by the equation:

$$Degree\ of\ unsharpness = \frac{Focus\ \times ORD}{FRD - ORD}$$

5

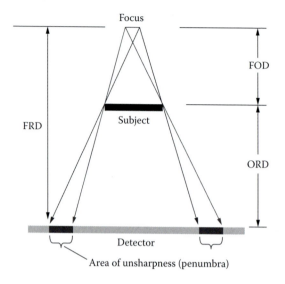

Figure 1.2 Diagram to demonstrate factors affecting geometric unsharpness.

To minimise geometric unsharpness (Figure 1.2)

- Fine focus should be used where possible.
- The object should be as close to the detector as possible (ideally in contact).
- The FRD should be as long as practicable as this minimises the penumbra.

n.b. Images with visible unsharpness are not diagnostic and need to be repeated.

Bucky/grids

Bucky assemblies/antiscatter grids are the most commonly used method to reduce noise, and thus improve contrast in an X-ray image in large body parts, e.g. spine and pelvis. This is achieved by absorbing scattered radiation, which is produced in all images. The grid allows a majority of the primary X-rays to be transmitted and a majority of the scattered X-rays to be absorbed. It is constructed from lead strips (which absorb most of the scatter) that are separated by a aluminium of fibrous material (**Figure 1.3**).

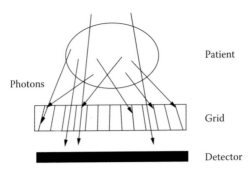

Figure 1.3 Application of a grid showing preferential absorptive of scatter.

The grid however, also absorbs some of the primary beam and the radiation exposure to the patient must be increased by a factor of 2–3 to compensate for the loss of primary and scattered X-rays removed by the grid. Grids can be stationary and simply placed between the patient and the image receptor or inserted into a bucky mechanism where they move in a reciprocating manner to absorb most of the scattered photons. Grids therefore increase the radiation dose to the patient.

The bucky is located under the X-ray table or vertical stand. The specifications of different grids can vary based on:

- The number of strips over the length of the grid (numbers of strips per centimetre).
- The grid ratio (height of the lead strips to the interspace distance).
- Whether the grid is focused or parallel (alignment of the lead strips). A focused grid allows more useful photons to reach the image detector, but has restrictions for the FRD used.
- The pattern of the lead strips or orientation.

The grid frequency can range from 30 to 80 lines/cm. The ratio can range from a ratio of 4:1 to 16:1. The higher the frequency or the ratio, the more the noise can be reduced by the effective removal of scatter. The grid pattern can be linear (strips running in one direction) or crossed (strips running perpendicular to one-another), where crossed grids are associated with higher noise reduction and higher patient doses.

The higher the grid capability to absorb scattered radiation (i.e. higher frequency or ratio or grid with crossed pattern), the more it absorbs useful X-ray photons and the more increase in exposure is needed. It is also important to note that grid misalignment may result in grid 'cut off' where a large number of useful X-ray photons are absorbed by the grid, thus causing a substantial loss of image density and the necessity to repeat the X-ray in most cases.

Resolution/definition

The resolution of any radiographic image can be measured objectively using a test tool. It is normally stated in line pairs per millimetre and, for a matrix size of 10 pixels/mm^2, there are approximately 5 lp/mm. If the image is assessed visually (subjectively), the ability to determine anatomy is referred to as 'definition'. Resolution and definition are both affected by all of the components of the digital image chain, as well as the geometry of the patient positioning. Definition (spatial resolution) is also affected by the characteristics of the detector and monitor, the pixel size and depth, the processing and display of the image (see Chapter 7, Image quality).

When assessing the diagnostic quality of an image, it may be better to measure definition, as the person viewing the image can assess if they can see structures within the image, e.g. joint space, bone trabeculae.

X-RAY DETECTORS

Ideally, all of the unscattered radiation leaving the patient should be absorbed by the imaging plate, and the scatter ignored by the detector. Unfortunately, this is not achievable. Digital detectors (photostimulable storage phosphor (PSP)) absorb up to 35 per cent of the transmitted beam and this may increase to 60 per cent with direct conversion digital systems. The remaining radiation passes through the detector and may again be scattered.

There are two main types of detector for conventional projection X-ray imaging: computed radiography (CR) and digital radiography (DR). Both use photostimulable phosphors and will be explained in more detail in Chapter 6, detective quantum efficiency (DQE) is often a measure that is quoted in order to make comparisons between various imaging systems.

IONISATION

This is the process of removing one or more of the electrons in an atom leaving the atom in an excited state or ionised. The remaining atom is then called an 'ion' and is positively charged as the electron is ejected. Ionisation is significant in a number of processes for image production. **Figure 1.4** demonstrates the process of ionisation.

Charged particles and photons of radiation are all able to ionise other atoms and the process features in the following instances:

- Production of X-rays in a tungsten target
  - Thermionic emission at the filament
  - Production of heat in a tungsten target
- Detection of radiation
  - Radiation measurement
  - Dosimetry of radiation effects
  - Fluoroscopy
  - Image production.
  - Radiation protection.

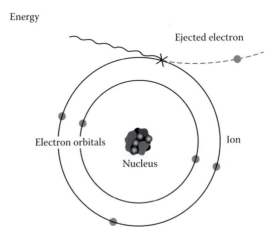

Figure 1.4 The process of ionisation.

DISPLAY SYSTEM AND VIEWING CONDITIONS

Images are viewed on visual display units (VDU). The image is a display of pixels (these are the smallest element of the image). The matrix size affects the spatial resolution of the image. All pixels within the digital images have been processed before they are displayed. A look-up table (LUT) is applied to each pixel and this enhances the contrast and dynamic range of the image. Data may be enhanced differently by applying a different LUT and an almost infinite number of variables can be used to manipulate the data to provide an optimum image. The images can also be manipulated post-acquisition by the operator to enhance various factors, e.g. contrast, brightness, or suppress factors, like noise.

RADIATION DOSE

It is a legal requirement (IRR'99) to record the radiation dose delivered to the patient. This will be discussed in Chapter 8. There are a number of ways used in practice, the simplest being noting down the exposures used and the room used. Alternatively, the diamentor(DAP) reading may be noted, alternatively some DR and fluoroscopy units state a dose reading. These methods give sufficient data to allow the radiation dose to the patient to be calculated at a later date using more sophisticated methods.

PRACTITIONER'S SKILL AND PERCEPTION

The concept and science of image perception is beyond the scope of this book, however, it should be noted that the practitioners viewing the image displayed on the monitor may see very different images.

There is research which clearly demonstrates that the experience and skill of the practitioner affects their ability to perceive pathology or abnormalities with the image.

MCQs

1. **Which of the following statements best describes 'image definition'**
   a. A subjective measurement
   b. Ability to resolve 5 lp/mm
   c. Ability to see a specific anatomical structure
   d. Diagnostic quality image.

2. **Scattered radiation can be described as:**
   a. X-rays produced by the X-ray tube
   b. Radiation absorbed by the patient
   c. X-rays which improve image quality
   d. Noise which does not convey useful information from the patient.

3. **You are producing an image of the spine. The focus receptor distance (FRD) is 100 cm and the spine is 20 cm from the imaging plane. The spine is 40 cm long. What is the length of the spine in the image?**
   a. 50 cm
   b. 48 cm
   c. 40 cm
   d. 20 cm.

4. **Which of the following factors will not enhance image quality?**
   a. Short ORD
   b. Long FRD
   c. Large focal spot
   d. Small focal spot.

5. **Which of the following abbreviations best describes the principle of radiation protection?**
   a. IR(ME)R
   b. ALARA
   c. ALARP
   d. IRR'99.

6. If the focus of the X-ray tube is 1 mm, the focus is 100 cm from the detector and the object is 1 cm from the detector calculate the unsharpness:
   a. 1 mm
   b. 0.1 mm
   c. 0.02 mm
   d. 0.01 mm.

7. You are producing an image of the finger. The FRD is 100 cm and the finger is 1 cm from the imaging plane. What is the magnification in the image?
   a. 0.9 times
   b. 0.5 times
   c. 1.1 times
   d. 1.01 times.

8. Which of the following statements best describes the function of a grid?
   a. The grid only removes scattered radiation.
   b. The grid only removes the primary beam radiation.
   c. The grid removes scattered radiation more efficiently than the primary beam.
   d. The grid removes both scattered and the primary beam as efficiently as each other.

9. The grid ratio is:
   a. The number of lead strips per centimetre
   b. The height of the lead strip to the height of the interspace
   c. The height of the lead strip to the thickness of the interspace
   d. The direction of the lead strips in relation to the primary beam.

10. Ionisation of atoms produces:
    a. Free electrons
    b. Ionised atoms
    c. Positive atoms
    d. All of the above.

CHAPTER 2
MATHEMATICS FOR MEDICAL IMAGING

INTRODUCTION

The aim of this chapter is to give the student an understanding of the basic principles of the mathematics underpinning diagnostic radiography. It is essential that any practitioner operating within an imaging department and using ionising radiation has a sound base for their knowledge. You need to comprehend the maths and be able to explain the factors affecting the production of diagnostic images, the principles of exposure manipulation and safety within X-ray departments.

Learning objectives
The student should be able to:
- State the base International System of Units (SI) units
- Explain the applied SI units for radiography
- Understand and explain the basic mathematical concepts used in radiography

BASIC MATHEMATICS

There are a number of basic tasks which all radiographers should be able to perform. Simple addition, subtraction, multiplication and division, for example, enable the student to manipulate exposure factors at different distances and calculate radiation dose.

Exposure calculations

The radiation output from an X-ray tube is a product of the current applied to the X-ray tube (measured in milliamps (mA)), the duration of the exposure (measured in seconds (s)) and also the voltage applied to the X-ray tube (measured in kilovoltage (kVp)).

Radiation output is normally known as the intensity of the X-ray beam and needs to be varied to enable different body parts to be imaged. Other factors affect the intensity of the radiation beam reaching the detector. These are:

- The energy of the beam
- The medium through which the beam passes
- The distances between the X-ray source, the patient and the detector
- If a grid or Bucky is used to eliminate scattered radiation
- The filtration applied to the X-ray tube.

When the radiographic technique needs to be modified either to change the distances between the elements or if the exposure time needs to be reduced, then a new exposure may need to be calculated. This can be done by using the following formula:

$$\frac{\text{mAs} \times \text{kV}p^4}{\text{grid factor} \times \text{FR}D^2} = \frac{\text{mAs} \times \text{kV}p^4}{\text{grid factor} \times \text{FR}D^2} \, .$$

The mAs and kVp, use of a grid and distance for the initial examination, are put into the left-hand side of the equation and the new ones into the right-hand side. Changing the mAs is straightforward as the intensity of the beam is directly proportional to the mAs. Changing the kVp is more complex and the calculation should be performed with the kVp to the fourth power, i.e. kVp^4. If no grid is used, the grid factor is 1, e.g. initial exposure: 1 mAs, 70 kVp, 150 cm focus receptor distance (FRD), grid factor 2. Question: What is the required mAs at 180 cm FRD, 70 kVp and grid factor 1?

$$\frac{1 \times 70^4}{2 \times 150^2} = \frac{\chi \times 70^4}{1 \times 180^2} \, .$$

The new exposure needs to be 1.62 mAs to account for the increased distance and the inverse square law.

International system of units

To standardise the units of measurement used in science, SI units are used within the scientific community. There are seven standard base units and these are listed in **Table 2.1**.

From these standard base units, other SI units may be derived which are more applicable to radiography for example. These derived SI units are defined in **Table 2.2** with their applications.

Measurement prefixes (powers)

There are a number of times in radiography when we use numbers which are either multiplications or fractions of the base units. These

Table 2.1 SI base units.

Base quantity	Name	Symbol
Length	metre	m
Mass	kilogram	kg
Time	second	s
Electric current	ampere	A
Temperature	kelvin	K
Amount of substance	mole	mol
Luminous intensity	candela	cd

Table 2.2 SI units used in radiography.

SI unit	Symbol	Definition of unit	Application
Joule (energy)	J	Ability to do work	Production of X-rays
Power	$J\,s^{-1}$	Rate of doing work	Output of the X-ray generator
Electric current	A (ampere)	Quantity of electrons flowing in an X-ray circuit. Usually expressed as the milliamperage (mA)	
Electrical potential	V (voltage)	Force which moves electrons around the X-ray circuit. Usually expressed as the maximum voltage applied across the X-ray tube (keV)	
Resistance	Ω (ohm)	The resistance of an electrical conductor	
	mAs	mA multiplied by the duration of the exposure	
Gray	Gy	Energy imparted to a body	Measures the absorbed radiation dose
Sievert	Sv	Dose in Grays × quality factor	Measures the biological effect of ionising radiation

can be expressed as indices, i.e. 10^2, which is shorthand for 10×10 or 100. If numbers are divided by 10s, the indices are minus numbers, i.e. 10^{-2} or one hundredth, e.g. kilovoltage and milliamps.

- The voltage which drives the electrons across the X-ray tube is measured in kilovolts (10^3 volts).
- The current used to produce a stream of electrons to the filament of the X-ray tube is measured in milliamps (10^{-3} of an amp).

The scale of values needed in radiography ranges from:

- tera as in 'terabytes' (TB) (10^{12} bytes or 1 billion bytes) to
- nano as in 'nanometre' (nm) (10^{-9} of a metre or 1 thousand millionth of a metre).

Other useful powers are:

- giga as in 'gigabecquerels' (Gbq) (10^9 becquerels or one thousand million becquerels)
- mega as in 'megahertz' (MHz) (10^6 hertz or 1 million hertz)
- centi as in 'centigray' (cGy) (10^{-2} Grays or 100th of a Gray)
- micro as in 'microgram' (µg) (10^{-6} gram or 1 millionth of a gram).

Multiplication and division of powers

If we need to multiply indices together, as long as the base is the same, we simply add the powers together, i.e. $10^2 + 10^2 = 10^4$ or 10 000; to divide, we turn the lower indices to a negative number and simply add again, i.e.

$$\frac{10\ 000}{100}$$

This becomes $10^4 + 10^{-2}$, which is 10^2 (100).

Logarithms (logs)

Before the invention of the calculator, there was a simple method of multiplying and dividing complex numbers. These were called common logarithms. Tables were used to convert numbers into indices and then the numbers were simply added or subtracted as above.

There are two important types of logs used in science:

1. Common logs or logs to the base 10
2. Natural logs (ln) or logarithms to the base e.

Natural logs are associated with exponential functions, such as the half value thickness or radioactive decay. Logarithmic scales are useful when displaying data graphically with a large range of values, e.g. 1 to 1 million. Exponential data displayed on a log scale will product a straight line rather than a curve.

Some computed radiography systems express the exposure index(EI) logrithmically and you need to be aware of the magnitude of change on this scale, e.g. if the expected EI is 2,

- a variation of +1 is 10 times the intended exposure;
- a variation of +0.3 is twice the intended exposure;
- a variation of −0.3 is half the intended exposure.

Graphs

A graph is a way of displaying data in a diagram. In its simplest sense, a graph can be used to display one set of data and its relationship against another. Alternatively, different data sets can be displayed to make visual comparisons. For example, see Chapter 4 and Chapter 5, where the graphs are used to display X-ray spectra.

There are occasions when a logarithmic scale is used to display scientific data in radiography, such as radioactive decay. Examples of the effect of a logarithmic scale when presenting the same data are shown in **Figure 2.1**.

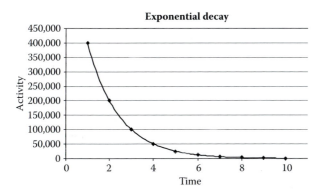

Figure 2.1 The effect of different scales on data display.

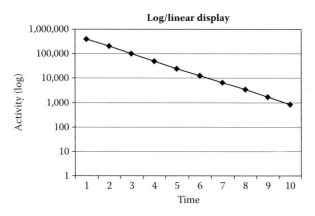

Figure 2.1 (continued)

Having the data represented by a straight line allows more accurate estimation of values between data points (interpolation) and points before or after the data measured (extrapolation).

Line focus principle

X-rays are produced when a fast-moving stream of electrons are decelerated by the target of the X-ray tube. The area bombarded by the X-rays is known as the focus. There are two conflicting variables when producing X-rays in an X-ray tube. These are:

- The focal area should be as large as possible to dissipate the heat produced.
- The apparent focus should be as small as possible by to produce sharp images.

These contradicting requirements are resolved as much as possible by the line focus principle. The focal track of the anode disc is angled at about 16–20° and forms the outer diameter of a large disc which may be up to 200 mm in diameter, whereas the apparent focus may be as small as 0.3 mm^2.

The relationship between the real focus and the apparent focus can be given by the equation:

$$a = r \sin \theta.$$

where a is the apparent focus, r is the real (actual) focus, θ is the angle of the anode. **Figure 2.2** demonstrates the relationship of the factors.

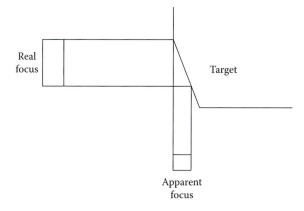

Figure 2.2 Line focus principle.

Similar triangles

It may be useful to practitioners to use similar triangles to calculate values used in radiography. Similar triangles can be used to calculate:

- The magnification of the image.
- The geometric unsharpness of the image.

If we consider the set up for imaging from Chapter 1 to demonstrate magnification, you can see there are two triangles of different sizes. Both triangles have the same internal angles, but one is bigger than the other. To calculate the length of any side of similar triangles, the ratio of the lengths is used (**Figure 2.3**). For example, if the lengths of two of the three sides are known, the size of the third can be calculated using ratios.

Inverse square law

The inverse square law is a mathematical way of calculating the intensity of an X-ray beam at differing distances from the X-ray tube output. It has important consequences for radiation protection and calculating the exposure factors needed when modifying radiographic techniques at different distances.

The inverse square law for radiation states:

The intensity of an X-ray beam is inversely proportional to the square of the distance.

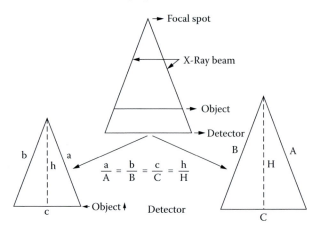

Figure 2.3 Similar triangles.

The law only applies if the radiation is from a point source, the radiation beam is homogenous and there is no attenuation between the source of radiation and the detector. None of these three conditions apply to an X-ray beam used for radiography. However, for practical purposes, the inverse square law may be generally applied to radiographic practice.

Practically, therefore, if the beam is measured at distances from a source of X-rays, the following applies:

- If the distance is doubled, the intensity falls to one-quarter of its original value.
- If it is trebled, the intensity falls to one-ninth.
- At four times the distance, it is 1/16, etc.

The formula is therefore:

$$I \propto \frac{1}{d^2} \, .$$

where I is intensity and d is distance. This may be represented as depicted in **Figure 2.4**.

In terms of radiation protection, the inverse square law demonstrates the effect of distance from a radiation source, e.g. X-ray tube or

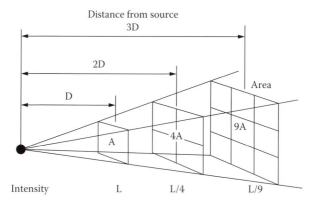

Figure 2.4 Inverse square law.

radioactive patient. Application of the inverse square law may be helpful in reducing radiation dose to staff.

Statistics

It may be necessary to collect, state, analyse and display data from groups (populations) in radiography. The simple expression of the mean (average), mode (most common), median (middle number) and range of values may be useful to calculate. Standard deviation may be used to demonstrate the variance from the mean. A low standard deviation indicates that the data points tend to be very close to the mean, whereas high standard deviation indicates that the data points are spread out over a wide range of values.

Descriptive statistics are used to summarise the population data by describing what was observed in the sample numerically or graphically. Inferential statistics uses patterns in the sample data to draw inferences about the population represented.

Statistical analysis may again be useful, and there are a number of common tests which may be used to analyse data:

- Analysis of variance (ANOVA)
- Chi-squared test
- Mann–Whitney U test
- *t*-test.

MCQs

1. **The voltage of an X-ray beam is conventionally measured in:**
   a. Joules per second
   b. kVp
   c. Joules
   d. mAs.

2. **One joule is equivalent to which of the following quantities?**
   a. $1 \, m^2 \, s$
   b. $1 \, N$
   c. $1 \, kg \, m^2 \, s^{-2}$
   d. $1 \, K \, m^2$.

3. **Which of the following is not an SI base unit?**
   a. Metre
   b. Second
   c. Kelvin
   d. Gray.

4. **If a radiographic image requires 20 mAs to produce the required density and the mAs was set at 200 mAs, what is the time setting?**
   a. 4 seconds
   b. 0.1 seconds
   c. 10 seconds
   d. 0.01 seconds.

5. **If the output of an X-ray tube is measured at 20 mGy at 100 cm, what will be the approximate output at 3 m?**
   a. 8 mGy
   b. 2.2 mGy
   c. 22 mGy
   d. 0.22 mGy.

6. **Using the formula a = r sin θ, calculate the size of the apparent focus if the anode angle is 17° and the real focus is 2 mm (sin 17° is 0.3)**
   a. 0.6 mm
   b. 2 mm
   c. 1.2 mm
   d. 0.22 mm.

7. **The SI unit of absorbed dose is the:**
   a. Milligray
   b. Gray
   c. Sievert
   d. Megagray.

8. **The SI unit of dose equivalent is the:**
   a. Milligray
   b. Gray
   c. Sievert
   d. millisievert.

9. **The SI unit of radioactivity is the:**
   a. Curie
   b. Rad
   c. Becquerel
   d. Coulomb.

10. **Ten to the power of 2 (10^2) is equivalent to:**
    a. 10
    b. 100
    c. 1000
    d. 10 000.

CHAPTER 3
PHYSICS FOR MEDICAL IMAGING

INTRODUCTION

The aim of this chapter is to introduce aspects of physics that are important within imaging science. These include; atomic structure, atomic number, mass number, electrons, elements, compounds, radioactivity, isotopes, principles of radioactive decay, work, energy, heat, transfer of heat, waves, sound, magnetism, electricity, electromagnetic radiation.

Learning objectives

The student should be able to:

- Explain atomic structure.
- Explain the principles of radioactivity and radioactive decay.
- Explain concepts of work, heat, waves and different forms of energy.
- Explain electromagnetic radiation and understand energy characteristics in respect of the electromagnetic spectrum.

THE ATOM

All matter within the universe is made from atoms.

Atomic structure

The simplest atom known is that of hydrogen, it consists of 2 sub-atomic particles; a proton and an electron. All other atoms have a 3rd sub-atomic particle known as a neutron.

Protons and neutrons form the nucleus of the atom and are known as nucleons. The electrons orbit the nucleus and are not attached directly to it. They are held in place primarily by the electrostatic force produced by the positively charged protons attracting the negatively charged electrons.

Protons: have a relative positive charge of +1 and relative atomic weight of 1. Although it is possible to examine the sub-structure of a proton in much more detail we will just mention quarks. The proton is composed of 2 up quarks and one down-quark.

Neutrons: DO NOT have a charge but have the same relative mass of 1. Apart from not having a net electric charge, neutrons do have a similar structure to protons and also contain quarks but this time the neutron is composed of one up-quark and two down-quarks.

Why talk about quarks? The reason we mention quarks is that they play a very important role in holding the nucleus together. As the protons in a nucleus all have a positive charge they naturally repel each other and try to separate the nucleus but it is thought that the arrangements of quarks produce very strong bonds to hold the nucleus together. These are referred to as the short range nuclear binding energy

Electrons: have a relative negative charge of –1 but have a mass 1840 times less than both protons and neutrons. Electrons are known as 'elementary particles,' which mean they do not have a sub-structure in the same way as protons and neutrons.

Figure 3.1 illustrates the arrangements of the sub-atomic particles, while the **Table 3.1** summarises them.

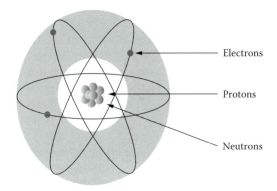

Figure 3.1 Arrangement of sub-atomic particles.

Table 3.1 SI Characteristics of the fundamental particles.

Summary table			
Sub-atomic particle	**Relative charge**	**Relative weight**	**Location**
Proton	+1	1	Part of the nucleus
Neutron	0	1	Part of the nucleus
Electrons	−1	1	Orbits the nucleus
		1840	

Atomic number

All atoms have a specific atomic number and this is based on the number of protons in the nucleus. For example, naturally occurring carbon has 6 protons forming part of its nucleus and therefore has an atomic number of 6.

Mass number

The mass number is the total number of protons and neutrons that form the nucleus. As electrons have negligible weight they are not included in the mass number. The commonest form of carbon consists of 6 protons and 6 neutrons and therefore has a mass number of 12. This natural form of carbon is referred to as 'carbon 12'.

Electrons and electron orbitals

The electrons in any atom 'orbit' the nucleus in energy bands called electron shells. If this did not happen the electrons would exist remotely from the nucleus and randomly within matter. Many aspects of modern physics, including the way X-rays are produced and interact with matter provide us with a strong indication that electron orbitals provide the most likely structural framework for those electrons which are bound to atoms. Everything about modern physics points to the existence of discrete energy bands each of which can contain a predictable maximum number of electrons.

- It is important to say at this stage that inner energy bands are the ones which fill up first and that if an electron is forcibly removed from an inner shell then another from a shell further away from the nucleus will move in to take its place.
- In making this transition however, the electron loses energy as it requires less energy to exist in a shell closer to the nucleus of an atom that in one further out.
- Each shell has within it, a whole series of sub-shells which have very slightly different energy values from each other, thus allowing the electrons to move about within their shells but without undergoing repeated collisions with each other. When considering electron shells it is always easiest in the early stages to consider the balanced atom where there are an equal number of electrons as there are protons (i.e. where the atomic number of the atom gives the number of electrons circulating in its energy shell or shells).
- The shells of the atom are commonly identified using letters, with the inner-most shell (that's the one nearest the nucleus) being the K shell and subsequent shells, (working away from the nucleus), being called L, M, N shells etc. When it comes to determining the maximum number of electrons in each shell then a different identification system has to be used. Now the K shell becomes shell number 1, the L shell is shell number 2 etc (see the table below). We can now apply a formula to determine the **maximum** electron capacity for each shell: If we take the n-value of the shell to be its identifying number then the maximum electron capacity per shell is given by the formula $2n^2$.

Table 3.2 shows the shells and electron capacity.

Table 3.2 Maximum number of electrons in shells.

Shell	Shell number	$2n^2$ value	Maximum no of electrons
K	1	2	2
L	2	8	8
M	3	18	18
N	4	32	32

The mean energy value of each shell is determined by the atomic number of the atom and this energy value is greatest for the innermost (k) shell, diminishing sequentially in shells further away from the nucleus. The level of attraction between the positive nucleus and the negatively charged electrons will determine how securely the electrons are bound into the atom. (See page 51 for tungsten atom with its orbitals.)

Binding Energy

The binding energy of an electron is that amount of energy which is required to remove the electron from its atom and such an event will leave an atom which has been ionised. It is worth noting that an electron so affected must, in the first place, have been bound into an atom (i.e. existed within an electron shell) and that this electron must be removed from the atom, not simply removed from its shell (which is an alternative process leading commonly to fluorescence). The binding energy of an electron is determined by:

a. the number of protons in the nucleus of the atom (i.e. its atomic number)
b. the proximity of any electron to its nucleus (i.e. the orbit it sits in).

Essentially the nucleus can be considered as a strong attractive force for electrons, especially in high atomic number materials where the nucleus contains larger numbers of positively charged protons. This should help to explain both a) & b) above.

■ You also need to understand though, that it is not possible for electrons to come to rest within the atom anywhere other than in the electron orbitals which explains why the electrons are not simply found 'glued' to the surface of the nucleus by the electrostatic forces which exist between the positively and negatively charged particles.

Every electron in any given shell of a specific atom will have the same binding energy. For example, the binding energy of K shell electrons in tungsten (W) is always 69.5keV and L shell electrons in tungsten always have a binding energy of 10.2keV. In short, the binding energy of any electron is not determined by the electron itself but rather, it is a function of the atomic number of the atom and the energy orbital (or shell) in which the electron exists.

Atomic symbols and the periodic table

Every atom known is included on a table known as the periodic table. Each type of atom has its own letters (symbol) accompanied by the atomic number and mass number.

If we consider carbon once again this will be written as:

$$\substack{(\text{mass number}) \\ (\text{atomic number})} \substack{12 \\ 6} C$$

This is also known as a 'nuclide'.

Atomic balance

You should think of the nucleus and the electron shells as being related, but separate from each other because it is very rare for natural events in daily life here on Earth to cause the electrons to enter the nucleus. Likewise, the **nucleons** (the collective name for protons and neutrons - because they exist in the nucleus) rarely move out of the nucleus.

In any given atom it is common for there to be the same number of electrons, collectively, within the electron shells as there are protons in the nucleus. This is known as an electrically balanced atom. But what happens if the nucleus and the electron shells become imbalanced electrically?

- if an atom gains an electron (which is a relatively common occurrence for some atoms), it is referred to as a negatively charged atom, also known as a negative **ion** or an **anion** (because it is attracted to a positive electrode or anode);
- if an atom loses an electron (again, relatively common) it leaves a positively charged atom, known as a positive ion or a **cation** (pronounced cat-ion), because it is attracted to a cathode.

An **ion** therefore is an atom in which there is an electrical imbalance between its nucleus and electron orbits.

In this atom, the nucleus is actually about 3,700 times heavier than the collective electrons circulating around it and therefore that nucleus contains far more than 99% of the mass of the atom.

Let's imagine that the atom was the size of an international rugby stadium. In such a scenario the nucleus of the atom, on the same scale, would be no bigger than a cherry (and the electrons would be smaller than pin heads). The nucleus is extremely dense $\left(\text{because density} = \frac{mass}{volume.}\right)$

Within physics most but not all stable atoms try to be in balance.

Ions

We mentioned before that atoms are normally electrically neutral with equal numbers of protons and electrons. It is possible for atoms to lose this balance and have a different number of electrons than protons resulting in a net positive or negative charge; it is then known as an ion.

Isotopes

Some atoms of the same element which have the same numbers of protons and electrons may have differing number of neutrons. These variations are called isotopes and have the same atomic number but a different atomic mass (Total of nucleons).

A good example of an atom with a number of isotopes is carbon, which has a total of 15 known isotopes. Carbon 12 is by far the commonest accounting for over 99% of all the carbon on earth. Three other well known isotopes of carbon are carbon 11, carbon 13 and carbon 14. These and other isotopes of carbon are unstable and undergo radioactive decay.

Elements

An element is quite simply a substance that only contains a single type of atom.

Compounds

A compound on the other hand is composed of more than one type of atom. Compounds can be quite different in the way they react when compared to the parent atoms and can have completely different properties. For example; common table salt is actually sodium chloride, we use this everyday in cooking and food preservation but if we look at the parent atoms they are very different. Sodium is actually explosive in water and highly volatile, while chlorine is a dense green poisonous gas.

RADIOACTIVITY

This is a random process associated with the nucleus of an atom. In its simplest term it is the break down in nuclear coherence and does NOT involve the electrons. As such it is not influenced by external environmental factors such as heat or pressure. This also means it can not be controlled or even predicted when considering individual atoms.

Principles of Radioactive Decay

As we said earlier, atoms naturally try to be in balance. Nuclear decay involves an unstable atom trying to become stable and balanced. In order for the atom to try and stabilise the nucleus undergoes some form of emission of particles and or charge, so that it can move to a more stable state.

There are three types of emission that occur:
1. Alpha particle emission (α - emission)
2. Beta particle emission (β - emission)
3. Gamma ray emission (γ - emission)

The unit of radioactivity is the Becquerel and is defined as: *1 disintegration per second.*

γ – emission and X-rays

γ rays are produced as a by product of either α or β decay. As the nucleus changes as a result these emissions it can result in the atom having excess energy. As the atom tries to become stable and balanced it has to dispose of this excess energy. The result is that monoenergetic photons of energy are emitted in the form of gamma radiation.

X-rays and γ radiation with the same energy and wavelength have identical properties ie an X-ray generated at 140kVp will be identical to γ radiation emitted by the decay of technetium 99mTc. The only way to distinguish them is their origins. γ radiation comes from the nucleus of the atom and X-ray are produced within the orbits of the atom.

Penetrating power of the emissions

Radioactive emissions have different power to penetrate materials. Alpha particles are highly ionising radiation and very destructive. Fortunately they are relatively big and heavy in atomic terms and can only travel a few centimetres in air and easily stopped even by a piece of paper.

Beta particles have a lower charge than alpha particles. The charge is not really high enough to directly cause ionisation but capable of breaking certain chemical bonds which may subsequently form ions.

Gamma radiation is a highly penetrating form of ionising radiation. They have a specific wavelength of γ radiation which can only have come from a specific atom undergoing radioactive decay.

FORCE, WORK, ENERGY AND POWER

Force: is defined as the ability to move a stationary body OR to increase/decrease the speed of a moving body.

It's unit of measure is the newton (N).

$$1 \text{ newton} = 1 \text{ kg x m/s}^2$$

The Newton is therefore the amount of force required to move a mass of 1kg at an acceleration rate of I meter per second, per second.

Work: Is effectively done if the object is moved. If a force of 1 newton was need to move an object over 1 metre then this would equate to 1 joule of work done.

The unit of measure is the joule (J).

$$1 \text{ joule} = 1 \text{ newton x } 1 \text{ metre}$$

Energy: Is effectively the same as work in that it equates to the ability to do work and uses the same unit of measure the joule.

However, it is quoted in two ways, potential and kinetic energy.

Potential Energy (PE) is the amount of energy which a body is capable of emitting.

Kinetic Energy (KE) is the amount of energy actually being used at the time, ie the work being done during the activity.

Power: Is derived by the rate at which energy is used.

It is measured in two ways either as joules per second or as watts, 1 joules per second (J/s) is the same as 1 watt (W).

HEAT

All atoms are in constant motion and because of this they possess kinetic energy. Heat as a form of energy is also measured in joules. Different materials such as solids, liquids or gases have slightly different amounts of motion depending on their chemical structure. This inherent motion is also affected by certain extrinsic factors. Anything that increases the amount of motion will lead to an increase in kinetic energy and effectively to an increase in temperature.

Transfer of Heat

There are 3 forms of heat transfer; conduction, convection and radiation.

Conduction

Requires the atoms to be very tightly packed together and as such is the dominant form of heat transfer for solids but conduction does occur in liquids and to a lesser extent even gases. As a material is heated the atoms within it start to vibrate more due to their increased energy state. Conduction occurs when this vibration starts to spread and pass heat energy to adjacent atoms. It is affected by certain physical characteristics such as the material density, its cross section and length as well as the temperature difference between adjacent points.

Convection

Heat transfer occurs when a current or flow of heat is created inside the material which is why it is restricted to liquids and gases. As a liquid or gas is heated the atoms tend to spread out due to the increase in their energy state this makes them less dense and they tend to rise and move away from the source of heat. As they move further away from the heat source they start to cool down become more dense and start to fall back down again. This forms a circular current called convection.

Radiation

This form of heat transfer is related to vibration of atoms in a similar way to the other forms of heat transfer. As the atoms are continuously heated and given energy they vibrate and as they do they give off pure energy as a wave which has both magnetic and electrical properties. This type of energy is part of the electro-magnetic spectrum known as infra-red radiation. As it is an electro-magnetic wave heat transfer does not require a medium and can even occur through a vacuum or void in space.

All atoms absorb and radiate heat by this method to some extent as all atoms are in constant motion, unless they are at absolute zero (0°Kelvin or -273°C) where all motion stops. Heat transfer is influenced by such things as the surface texture and colour of the material involved and at its most efficient is called black body radiation.

WAVES

Waves allow energy, such as electrical, magnetic or sound, to travel or transfer from one point to another and so on through any form of medium.

A good analogy is to imagine how a wave is created by lots of people in football stadium. Everyone in the ground sits down to begin with then one person stands up, then the person next to them stands up, the first person sits back down again and the 3rd person now stands up, the second sits down the 4th stands up and so on, before long this movement has travelled all the way around the stadium. The people themselves are still in the same seats but energy has travelled all the way around the stadium. This is essentially how energy is transferred.

Waves have three main components; amplitude, frequency and speed. The amplitude is the height of the wave while the frequency relates to how quick it switches between its lowest and highest points, while its speed is obviously how far it travels in a certain time. In our analogy the

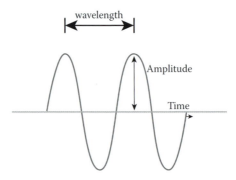

Frequency is the number of wavelengths
passing a point
Velocity is frequency x wavelength

Figure 3.2 Shows the parts of a sine wave.

amplitude is how high people in the crowd stand up, the quicker they stand up and down the higher the frequency of the wave. While the speed is how quickly this movement travels around the stadium. The length of the wave is also important (wavelength) and may be defined as the distance over which the wave repeats itself **(Figure 3.2)**.

Waves generally travel in straight lines but they can be reflected, deflected, amplified or absorbed. Waves of energy can also interfere with each other. If we consider two sound waves heading towards each other if they cross at the point where both waves happen to be at their peak the waves will be added together and effectively amplified.

SOUND

Sound is created by a vibrating object that causes compression and decompression pressure to build within a medium in sync with the vibration. This creates a longitudinal pressure wave which flows away from the vibrating object.

If the pressure wave travels towards the human ear it causes a vibration of the ear drum at the same frequency as the source and if the frequency falls somewhere between 20 Hertz (20 cycles per second) and 20 Kilohertz KHz) we perceive this as sound. Vibrations still occur outside this frequency range and strike the ear drum in the same way, it is simply that it falls outside the frequency range we are sensitive to.

Ultrasound is used in diagnostic imaging and uses sound above the audible range of 20 KHz and are usually between 2 and 18 Megahertz (MHz).

MAGNETISM

We are all familiar with a basic magnet, one that has a north and south pole. The basic law of magnetism states that like poles repel each other and opposite poles attract.

Inside the magnet there are a series of much smaller bits known as domains which have a north and south pole. In a non magnetic material these domains are randomly arranged so the material does not have a net magnetic force as all the magnetic forces cancel each other out. If on the other hand we do have a magnetic material it's domains are arranged so they line up with their north and south poles in the same direction.

Around this magnet are what is known as 'lines of magnetic flux energy', which form relatively large loops flowing between the north and south poles (Figure 3.3).

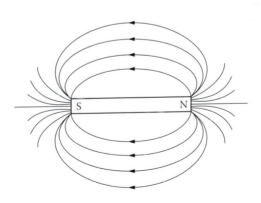

Figure 3.3 Lines of magnetic flux.

Magnetic Resonance Imaging MRI makes use of the property of nuclear magnetic resonance (NMR) to image nuclei of atoms inside the body. This provides excellent soft tissue images of the body.

ELECTRICITY AND ELECTRIC CHARGE

Electrical charge is related to the number of electrons in relation to the number of protons in a material. If these are the same then there is no net electrical charge. If we have more protons than electrons we effectively get a net positive charge overall and if we have more electrons than protons we have a small net negative charge. Like charges repel each other and unlike charges attract each other. Electricity is a flow of electrons within a conductor.

Electrical circuit

Electricity is a flow of electrons around a circuit and is called a current. If a potential difference is applied in an electrical circuit it will cause a current to flow. The positive electrode in a circuit is known as the anode and the negative the electrode the cathode. Electrons will flow from the negative electrode to the positive one providing there is a potential difference and the circuit is closed. Electrical conductors have a liberal supply of electrons loosely bound in their outer conduction shell. Silver is the best metal electrical conductor but copper is commonly used due to the expense. Both atoms have 1 electron in their conduction band.

Electrical insulators have all their electrons firmly bound to its molecules. In an insulating material it is much more difficult to disrupt the electrons and they usually break down before the electrons can flow. Good insulators are oil, plastics and rubber.

The SI unit of electric current is the Ampere (A). The ampere (amp) may be defined in a number of ways but the most suitable is:

1 amp is 1 Coulomb of charge flowing per second.

Power in an electrical sense can be determined from the current (amps) and voltage (volts). The power of an electrical circuit for X-ray production is measured in kilowatts (kW).

Electricity flows through the circuit in a number of forms which are relevant in radiography. These are:

- direct current (flows in one direction)
- alternating current flows in either directions depending on the potential difference.

ELECTROMAGNETIC RADIATION

This is a form of energy that is composed of both electrical and magnetic fields and travels through space as a wave.

As such it can be measured and classified by its wavelength and frequency. The electromagnetic spectrum includes radio waves, microwaves, infrared radiation, visible light, ultraviolet radiation, X-rays and gamma rays **(Figure 3.4)**.

Different types of electromagnetic radiation (EMR) carry energy at different frequencies and wavelengths and this dictates their properties (see spectrum above). All EMR travel in a vacuum at the speed of light (3×10^8 m/s) and travel in straight lines. They comprise of transverse variations of electrical & magnetic fields. (i.e. a transverse wave) All EMR carry energy and are not affected by electrical / magnetic

Electromagnetic Waves

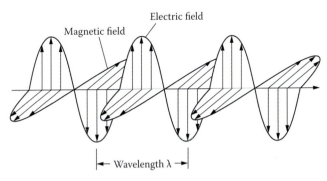

The wave is travelling in this direction

Figure 3.4 Electromagnetic spectrum.

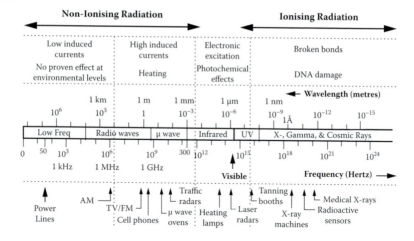

Figure 3.5 Electromagnetic spectrum.

fields. As the wavelengths shorten this leads to an increasing likelihood that they will interact with the atom causing ionisation.

These EMR are known as ionising radiation and this is particularly important within radiography with both X and Gamma rays directly interacting with the atoms within the body and causing ionisation **(Figure 3.5)**.

MCQs

1. **If we consider carbon written as follows:**

$$^{12}_{6}C$$

   Which statement is true? The atoms have:
   a. 12 protons and 6 neutrons and 6 electrons
   b. 6 protons, 6 neutrons and 6 electrons
   c. 6 protons and 6 neutrons and 12 electrons
   d. 12 protons and 6 neutrons and 6 electrons

2. **Which statement best describes electrons**
   a. Negative charge with an atomic weight of 1
   b. No charge with an atomic weight of 1
   c. Positive charge with an atomic weight of 1
   d. Negative charge with an atomic weight of $1/1840^{th}$ that of a proton
   e. positive charge with an atomic weight $1/1840^{th}$ that of a proton.

3. **Which statement best describes elements?**
   a. Elements are made of one type of atom
   b. Water H_2O is an example of an element
   c. They consist of different types of atoms
   d. All compounds are included on the periodic table.

4. **Which statement best describes an isotope?**
   a. Is an atom with less or more neutrons than protons.
   b. Is an atom with less or more electrons than protons.
   c. Is an atom with either a net negative or positive charge.
   d. Always undergoes radioactive decay.

5. **How would you define radioactivity?**
   a. The breakdown in nuclear coherence causing the ejection of an electron.
   b. Directly influenced by heat and temperature.
   c. Not influenced by external environmental factors such as heat or pressure and does NOT involve the electrons.
   d. Not influenced by external environmental factors such as heat or pressure and involves the ejection of electrons.

6. **Radioactive emissions have different ability to penetrate materials. Alpha particles are?**
   a. Relatively big and heavy in atomic terms and a highly ionising form of radiation able to penetrate the skin
   b. Relatively big and heavy in atomic terms and a highly ionising form of radiation but not able to penetrate the skin
   c. Relatively small and light but able to penetrate the skin
   d. Relatively small and light but unable to penetrate skin.

7. **Waves have three main components; amplitude, frequency and speed. The amplitude is:**
   a. Is the height of the wave
   b. How quick it switches between it's lowest and highest points
   c. Its velocity
   d. The number of waves per second.

8. **Electrical charge is present if:**
   a. There are more neutrons than electrons resulting in a net positive charge overall
   b. There are more protons than neutrons resulting in a net positive charge overall

   c. There are more protons than electrons resulting in a net positive charge overall

   d. There are more electrons than protons resulting in a net positive charge overall.

9. **Electromagnetic radiation is:**

   a. Radiation that has relatively long wavelengths much larger than an atom.

   b. Radiation that has relatively short wavelengths, much smaller than an atom.

   d. Radiation that has a wavelengths that is of a similar size to that of the atom.

   c. Radiation that the wavelength varies according to the frequency.

10. **Electromagnetic radiation is:**

   a. Classified only by its wave length

   b. Classified only by its frequency

   c. Classified by both its frequency and wavelength

   d. Always visible.

CHAPTER 4

X-RAYS, X-RAY TUBE AND X-RAY CIRCUIT

INTRODUCTION

It is essential that any practitioner understands the properties of X-rays and the way in which they are produced. The ability to generate a varied X-ray beam is necessary to produce diagnostic images with optimum a quality and minimum dose. The circuitry of the X-ray tube coverts a mains supply of 415 volts and 13 amps to the range of kilovolts (kV) and tube currents (mA) required to generate a range of X-rays. The circuitry allows an electrically safe process and facilitates exposure times from milliseconds to several seconds. The X-ray tube not only produces a beam of X-rays, but also dissipates the heat produced as a byproduct of the process efficiently, so repeated exposures can be made. It also needs to be electrically safe at the high voltages used.

Learning objectives

The student should be able to:

- Explain the properties of X-rays, the basic X-ray circuit and the range of exposure values generated.
- Understand and explain how electron interactions generate X-rays and the spectra produced.
- Explain and illustrate how changes to exposure factors and X-ray tube settings will affect the spectral output of X-rays.
- Explain how a significant amount of heat is dissipated following X-ray production.

X-RAYS

X-rays are invisible, cannot be heard, have no odour and are not affected by electric or magnetic fields. They are a form of electromagnetic radiation and have wavelengths in the range of 0.01 to 10 nanometres. X-rays are commonly referred to as 'photons' and have the ability to ionise other substances, i.e. they cause the atoms through which they pass to eject electrons from their electron shells. This ability accounts for imaging properties and their potential harmful effect. The ejected eloctrons can be absorbed and scattered in different media.

X-rays can be detected by their ability to ionise other substances, cause fluorescence, give rise to colour changes in several substances and produce changes which can be made visible in photographic film.

X-RAY TUBE

This book will only outline rotating anode X-ray tubes as this arrangement accounts for the majority of X-ray equipment. Stationary anode X-ray tubes have low ratings (heat capacity) and are now only found in dental equipment and small portable machines. An X-ray tube consists of two components:
1. The insert which is evacuated and is where the X-rays are produced.
2. The tube shield which supports the insert and is responsible for electrical and radiation safety.

The function of the X-ray tube is to:
- Provide a beam of X-rays from as near a point source as possible (focus).
- Dissipate the heat produced effectively to prevent damage to the X-ray tube (approximately 99 per cent of the energy conversions produce heat).
- Provide a consistent quality (kVp) and quantity (mAs) of radiation.

- Allow X-rays to emerge only from the window (port) of the housing of the tube and exclude emissions from elsewhere in the housing, which is lined with lead sheet.
- Provide an electrically safe environment for the practitioner.
- The tube is securely supported, but capable of easy movement into any position and then being maintained in that position.

There are numerous materials used in the construction of the X-ray tube and tube shield. These include:

- Tube housing – steel construction lined with lead (except port)
- Port – plastic or beryllium
- Insulation between the housing and insert – mineral oil
- Insert – nowadays these are made from metal/ceramics, but historically were made from borosilicate glass
- Filament (cathode) assembly/focusing cup – nickel or stainless steel
- Filament – tungsten
- Anode disc – molybdenum alloy or graphite disc or tungsten (90 per cent) and rhenium (10 per cent) alloy focal track with graphite backing
- Anode stem – molybdenum
- Stator windings – copper
- Additional filtration – aluminium and sometimes copper.

Figure 4.1 (a, b) shows a schematic diagram of the X-ray tube and a photograph showing the X-ray tube in its housing.

Parts of the X-ray tube

Insert (envelope)

This insert maintains a vacuum for X-ray production and contains the anode assembly and cathode assembly. Nowadays, metal/ceramics have replaced the borosilicate glass envelope as the metal component can be earthed so that there is no build up of static. The cathode and anode assemblies are fixed within the envelope and the envelope also supports these two electrodes in correct alignment at the correct distance. All seals and metal poles are carefully chosen to match the expansion coefficients of the different parts which will reduce the risk of damage to the insert during operation. Having the potential of +75 kv and –75 kv allows a maximum of 150 kV to be used. **Figure 4.2** illustrates the alignment and constituents of the tube insert.

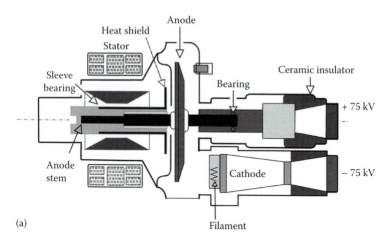

(a)

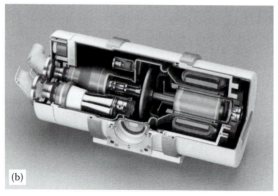

(b)

Figure 4.1 (a) X-ray tube and (b) housing.

Anode assembly

The anode assembly consists of:

- Anode disc and focal track
- Anode stem
- Rotor assembly
- HT connection for the positive side of the tube circuit.

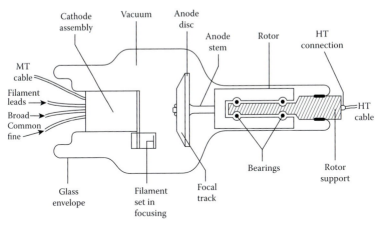

Figure 4.2 Tube insert.

The rotating anode consists of a tungsten rhenium disc which is typically 90–150 mm in diameter. A large rotating disc increases tube rating and thermal capacity. It may be a composite disc with a tungsten/rhenium focal track and a graphite or molybdenum backing which reduces the overall mass and acts as a heat sink.

The disc has a bevelled edge which forms the anode angle and focal track. The cathode focuses the electron beam on to the focal track where X-rays are produced (**Figure 4.3**). Typical angles for rotating X-ray tubes are between 16 and 20°.

The anode is attached to a molybdenum stem which connects it to the rotors. The anode stem has a small cross-section and is as long as possible in order to restrict the conduction of heat to the bearing assembly (*Note*: Molybdenum is a metal, so is an excellent conductor of heat). Heat conduction is restricted by the size and shape of the stem, not the material. The stem is connected to the copper rotor assembly. The rotors use induction via the stator windings to rotate the anode at speeds of 3000–9000 r.p.m. during exposures.

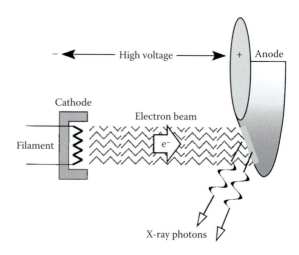

Figure 4.3 Cathode focusing the electron beam on to the anode angle where X-rays are produced.

Filament circuit

The filament circuit provides a circuit to the filament to facilitate thermionic emission of electrons. Changing the mA varies the current so that the temperature varies. As the mA increases, the number of electrons increases proportionally to the temperature.

Cathode assembly (filament)

The cathode assembly consists of:
- The filaments (fine and broad)
- Focusing cup which is negatively charged
- Electrical supply and connections:
  - Filament supply
  - HT supply to the negative side of the X-ray tube circuit

The purpose of the cathode is to produce thermionic emission of electrons which can be focused on and attracted to the anode. Thermionic emission is achieved by supplying a variable mA which heats the filament. The filament is a tightly coiled wire and increasing the mA causes increases in the temperature of the filament and hence

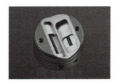

Figure 4.4 Focusing cup and foci.

the number of electrons in the electron cloud. Doubling the mA from 100 to 200 doubles the number of electrons and hence is directly proportional to the number of X-rays produced.

Focusing cup

The filament is encased in a nickel housing which focuses the electrons on to the focal track of the anode. This is achieved by having sharp edges to the focusing cup, which become negatively charged when the tube voltage is applied. The sharp edge concentrates the negative charge and this narrows the electron beam directed towards the anode. **Figure 4.4** shows the arrangement for fine and broad focus.

X-RAY CIRCUIT

The function of the X-ray circuit is to:
- Provide an electrically safe environment for the production of X-rays:
  - The housing is connected to earth via the high tension cables.
  - Live wires are electronically insulated.
  - The high tension and filament circuits are isolated from the mains supply.
- Provide a stable voltage to the autotransformer which is electronically isolated from the mains supply. This allows for a non-fluctuating supply of electricity to the components of the circuit.
- Modify the mains supply of 415 volts alternating current (ac) to a unidirectional current at voltages ranging from 28 to 150 kVp (high tension (HT) supply).

- Provide heat to the filament circuit. This creates thermionic emission to produce electrons at the anode of in the X-ray tube.
- Supply accurate and consistent control of the duration of the exposure from 0.001 seconds to several seconds (timer circuit).

The interaction of high-energy electrons with matter

Electrons released from the filament of the X-ray tube by thermionic emission are accelerated across the X-ray tube towards the target (anode) by the potential difference between the cathode and the anode.

- The number of electrons released in each exposure is determined by the selected mA.
- The kinetic energy acquired by the electrons is determined by the selected kV (or more accurately, keV).

As the electrons reach the tungsten target of the X-ray tube, they will start to undergo sub-atomic interactions with the atoms in the target.

Essentially three types of interaction will occur:

1. Incoming electrons with outer-shell electrons of the target atoms
2. Incoming electrons with inner-shell electrons of the target atoms
3. Incoming electrons with nuclei of the target atoms.

Incoming electrons will undertake many interactions (probably around 1000) with the target atoms before giving up all their kinetic energy. These interactions are most likely to occur within 0.5 mm of the surface of the target.

Interactions between incoming electrons and outer-shell electrons in tungsten

Tungsten has an atomic number of 74 and therefore there are (usually) 74 electrons in each atom of the target material available for interaction. The majority of those electrons will be in outer orbitals of each of the tungsten atoms and therefore the incoming electrons will require relatively small amounts of energy to interact with the shell-bound electrons as they are less tightly bound to the atom. **Figure 4.5** shows the atomic arrangement of tungsten.

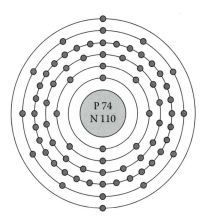

Figure 4.5 Tungsten atom demonstrating the number of electrons in the outer shells. P, protons; N, neutrons; •, electron; electron shells 2, 8, 18, 32, 12, 2, Corresponding to the K,L,M,N,O,P orbits.

Interactions producing heat

As the incoming electrons interact with the electrons in tungsten atoms (millions of times during each X-ray exposure), small amounts of energy are given up as electromagnetic radiations (EMR) due to the electrostatic repulsion which occurs between the two negatively charged sub-atomic particles.

The small amounts of energy released during each interaction are far too small to produce X-rays and virtually all of the energy is released as heat. As the greater proportion of the target material (in terms of volume) occurs in the outer orbitals of each tungsten atom, it follows that large proportions of the energy provided by the incoming electrons will be converted into EMR energies at the lower end of the spectrum – most commonly infrared energy (heat).

Each of the incoming electrons can undergo many thousands of these low energy-release interactions before coming to rest, making it very easy to understand how up to 99 per cent of the energy produced at the target of the X-ray tube occurs in the form of heat.

Interactions producing X-rays

X-rays are produced in the X-ray tube by two interactive processes between incoming electrons and the atoms of the target:

1. Characteristic radiation
2. Bremsstrahlung

Interactions between incoming electrons and inner-shell electrons in tungsten (characteristic X-ray production)

It is normal to consider K and L shells as inner shells or orbitals for the purposes of this description. These are the only two shells in tungsten where the ejection of an electron could lead to the emission of a photon of EMR which would both be X-rays in nature and also have sufficient energy to escape from the X-ray tube.

Two interactions are possible:

1. Excitation: where sufficient energy is given to the bound electron to raise it to the next orbital
2. Ionisation: where the binding energy of the orbital electron is overcome and it is released from the atom

Where **excitation** occurs, the electron which was removed from its shell has only been removed temporarily. It still remains within the structure of the atom and will ultimately return to its original position, giving out a photon of EMR with an energy equivalent to that acquired by the electron in raising itself to a different shell (or valence band). If the electron transition away from its shell and back again takes less than 10^{-14} seconds, then the process is known as 'fluorescence'; if it takes longer, it is known as 'phosphorescence'.

In addition to the possible production of characteristic radiation, both ionisation and excitation will also give rise to some heat production as energy is transferred to the target material during both processes but no X-rays will be produced.

In the case of **ionisation**, the released electron is known as a delta-ray and carries with it kinetic energy donated during the interaction. The delta-ray will go on to interact with other atoms until it has lost its acquired kinetic energy at which point it becomes indistinguishable from other electrons in the material.

It must be noted that ionisation can only occur in this way if the kinetic energy carried by the incoming electron (i.e. the keV applied across the X-ray tube) is equal to or greater than the specific binding energy of the orbital-bound electron. In the case of tungsten, the K-orbital binding energy is 69.5 keV and the L-orbital binding energy is given as 10.2 keV.

Ionisation of a K-shell electron will leave the atom with a vacancy in this orbital which cannot be sustained in nature. Immediately an electron from a shell further from the nucleus will drop into the K-shell and in doing so a photon of EMR will be released whose value equals the difference in binding energies between the receiving shell (the K-orbital here) and the 'donating' shell (**Figure 4.6**).

If we consider this process in tungsten, then the removal of a K-orbital electron would have arisen from the interaction of one of the shell-bound electrons with an incoming electron which carried with it a kinetic energy of at least 69.5 keV. There would then be a 'gap' in the K-orbital which, if filled by an L-orbital electron from within the atom, would give rise to a photon of EMR with energy of 59.3 keV (K-orbital binding energy (69.5 keV) minus L-orbital binding energy (10.2 keV)).

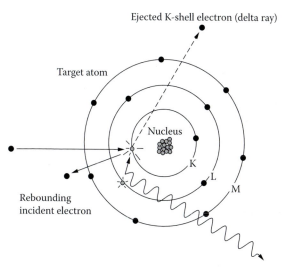

Figure 4.6 Diagram of the process of characteristic radiation.

A photon of EMR with energy of 59.3 keV would fall well within the X-ray region of the electromagnetic spectrum and would be known as a 'K-alpha emission'.

It is entirely possible that the vacancy in the K-orbital in the example above could be filled with an electron arising from the M-orbital. In such a case, the energy of the emission arising from the interaction would equal the difference in binding energies between the K-orbital electron (69.5 keV) and the M-orbital electron (2.5 keV), i.e. approximately 67 keV. This emission would be known as a K-beta X-ray photon.

It should be clear at this stage that irrespective of the energy of the incoming electron, provided that energy is greater than the binding energy of the shell-bound electron, removal of that electron will always lead to the production of X-rays which fall into well-defined energy bands. These radiations are characteristic of the material in which they are produced and their energy bands depend on three variables:

1. The atom type, i.e. the atomic number of the material which, in turn, determines the binding energies of the shells.
2. The shell from which the electron was ejected (e.g. K, L, M) for any given atom.
3. To a lesser extent, the shell from which the 'replacement' electron comes.

Characteristic line spectra are always produced by this process alongside the continuous spectra, as demonstrated in **Figure 4.7**. From an analysis point of view, the identity of every material can be determined by identifying its emission spectra (X-ray spectroscopy). More to the point, useful X-rays can be produced using this process, providing the target material has a high enough atomic number and the tube voltage is above 70 KeV.

It should be noted that characteristic radiation in any inner shell will not be produced alone. Wherever a K-alpha series of characteristic radiations is produced in tungsten, there will always be an L-series of emissions and an M-series of emissions (through to the last shell). The process works on a cascade basis, so that any gaps which appear in any shell are filled immediately to maintain the orbital stability of the atom.

A beam from characteristic X-ray production is called a homogenous beam. For tungsten K-shell emission, it gives a:

(a)

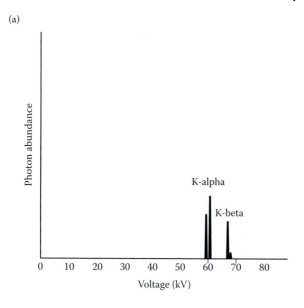

(b)

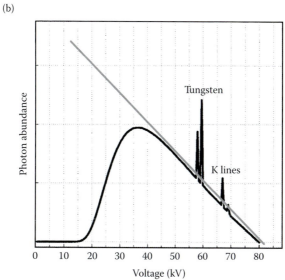

Figure 4.7(a) Characteristic radiation **(b)** Bremsstrahlung with characteristic radiation.

55

- 59.3 keV energy line (K-alpha)
- 67 keV energy line (K-beta).

Interactions between incoming electrons and the nucleus of the atom (Bremsstrahlung X-ray production)

This interaction process occurs when one electrically charged particle (in this case the incoming electron from the filament with its small negative charge) and large kinetic energy is deflected by a second charged mass (the nucleus of the tungsten atom which has a mass many thousands of times greater than the mass of the incoming electron, and a much greater (positive) charge also) (**Figure 4.8**).

The deflection will cause a change in momentum for the incoming electron which, in turn, gives rise to the emission of a photon of EMR. The loss of energy causes the incoming electron to slow down and therefore the common name for this process of X-ray production is the Bremsstrahlung process (meaning 'braking radiation' in German).

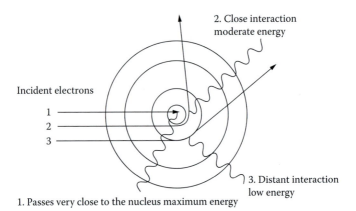

Figure 4.8 Diagram of the process of Bremsstrahlung.

The amount of kinetic energy given over to the photon of EMR (which is in the X-ray part of the electromagnetic spectrum) from the incoming electron is determined by how close the electron passes to the nucleus. The closer the electron passes to the nucleus, the greater will be the deflection experienced by it and the greater will be the loss of energy from the electron as a quantum of radiation. The exact energies of the various quanta produced in each X-ray exposure may be many and various from very low energy photons (which are completely absorbed by the X-ray tube) right through to interactions where the total energy of the incoming electron is given up. Therefore, as each interaction is likely to produce slightly different results from those of neighbouring interactions, the graphical representation, which is produced as a result of the activation of an X-ray tube, will demonstrate a range of X-ray energies being produced rather than the single-energy spectra found with characteristic X-ray production.

The graph in **Figure 4.7** is effectively a line chart which delineates an area underneath the graph. It is this whole area (underneath the line) which represents the total X-ray energy found in the beam and this enables the graph or X-ray spectrum to be used to compare beam outputs when exposure factors and other parameters are changed.

- A beam from Bremsstrahlung which is composed of a range of energies is known as a 'heterogeneous beam'.
- The only definite fixed point to be found on a graph representing the X-ray spectrum for the Bremsstrahlung process is the upper energy point (E_{max}). This is determined by the generating voltage applied across the X-ray tube (in keV) and therefore the kinetic energy carried by each of the incoming electrons.
- If the generating voltage is set at 100 keV, for example, then no electron can give up more than that amount of energy as it interacts with the nucleus of the target atom. It is found that some (though very, very few) incoming electrons do give up all of their energy in a single interaction with the charged nucleus. The energy of the photon of radiation produced would equal that amount of energy acquired by the electron as it accelerated towards the target of the X-ray tube and, which was then released in the interaction with the target atom – in our example above that would be 100 keV.

- Many incoming electrons will give up a proportion of their energy in an interaction with the nucleus of a target atom and, having done so, carry on through the target material to undergo further interactions (some of which will produce X-rays, but many more of which will produce yet more unwanted heat).
- **Figure 4.7** demonstrates that many of the Bremsstrahlung interactions produce X-rays which, as a proportion of the maximum possible photon energy, occur at about one-third to one-half of that energy. This is represented as the peak intensity of the beam of X-ray energies. The peak intensity of X-ray energies is also known as the kVp (kV-peak) and the relationship between keV and kVp can be confusing for students.
- The kVp for a given beam is numerically the same as the keV applied as the generating voltage across the X-ray tube during any given exposure. As an example, if the X-ray beam is generated with a tube voltage of 60 keV, then the peak energy output from the resulting X-ray beam will be 60 kVp. If you check this out on a 60 keV spectrum, it will be clear that the keV and the kVp do not occur at the same point on the energy axis of the graph. As stated above, the kVp will have an energy which is between one-third and one-half of the keV. Thus, although the two values are the same numerically, they are not the same.
- It is convenient to consider the beam output from the X-ray tube as being comparable to the input voltage used to generate the beam and this can be done easily if the numbers are the same. Perhaps the easy way to understand what is happening is to consider the keV as the energy which is put into the X-ray tube to produce a similar kVp output value. The difference in actual energy between the two values is utilised in the inevitable production of heat, which always accompanies the production of X-rays.

It must be noted that this graph shows the Bremsstrahlung spectrum of emissions for the X-radiations which escape the X-ray tube only. In reality, the X-ray beam produced at the surface of the target would show as a straight line graph with the beam intensity increasing as the beam energy decreased (grey line in graph). However, much of the low energy radiation is attenuated by the X-ray tube components and never escapes the tube complex itself.

X-RAY SPECTRA AND FACTORS AFFECTING THE QUALITY AND INTENSITY OF THE X-RAY BEAM

This section will consider the factors which influence the intensity and quality of the X-ray beam produced by the Bremsstrahlung process. First, there are a number of factors associated with a Bremsstrahlung curve which we must consider. The key thing to remember here is that:

- The quality of the radiation measures the beam's overall energy.
- The intensity is a measure of the number of X-ray photons.

The intensity of the beam represents the quantity of radiation produced at a given energy and the maximum beam intensity for the full range of energies which make up the heterogeneous beam is given by the curve on the Bremsstrahlung graph. Radiation intensity is a measure of the number of photons in a beam of a given cross-sectional area. The height of the Bremsstrahlung curve will be directly proportional to the intensity of the X-ray beam. This can be referred to as the size of the curve.

The quality of the X-ray beam measures how readily the beam will penetrate any given material (often measured using thicknesses of aluminium for a diagnostic X-ray beam). The half-value thickness of a beam of radiation is that amount of a given material which will attenuate 50 per cent of the intensity of the X-ray beam. Although the measure of half-value thickness can only strictly be used with homogenous (monochromatic) X-ray beams, it will provide a useful guide to the penetrating power of a heterogeneous (Bremsstrahlung) beam also. The quality of any beam of X-rays is proportional to its half-value thickness for any given material. With reference to the Bremsstrahlung curve, the energy of the beam is directly related to the position of the curve along the energy axis, i.e. a higher energy beam will be represented by the peak of the Bremsstrahlung curve being moved to the right along the energy (x) axis. This can be referred to as the shape of the curve.

The maximum beam energy is often referred to as E-max and is represented by the point at which the Bremsstrahlung curve's high energy point crosses the x-axis. For the purposes of the diagnostic X-ray beam, E-max will always be equal to the generating voltage (keV) of the particular X-ray beam.

Impact of changing the mA

The mA is a measure of the current flowing across the X-ray tube, often called the 'tube current'. Current in electrical terms is the flow of electrons (caused by a potential difference between the cathode and the anode) and its value in mA is determined by the number of electrons flowing per unit time. If the tube current is doubled from 200 to 400 mA, then there will be twice as many electrons making up the tube current and flowing across the X-ray tube.

Since each electron will be subjected to exactly the same potential difference, it will have exactly the same chance of creating an X-ray photon. Therefore, doubling the mA will double the number of X-rays produced but will not affect the energy range of the X-rays. The opposite would happen if the mA were halved (**Figure 4.9**). (E-max, the minimum energy value and the position of the peak of the curve across the graph will all remain the same.)

It can therefore be deduced that:
- Beam intensity is proportional to mA.
- Beam quality is unaffected by changes in mA.

Impact of changing the kV

The X-ray tube voltage (measured in keV) determines the potential difference between the cathode and the anode of the X-ray tube. This in turn will determine the kinetic energy acquired by each of the electrons as the current flows across the X-ray tube.

As the keV is increased, the speed at which the electrons impact on the target anode is also increased, which means that there are more opportunities for the conversion of the energy into X-rays (and also heat unfortunately). As more energy is available in the interaction process at the anode, the following events will all occur:

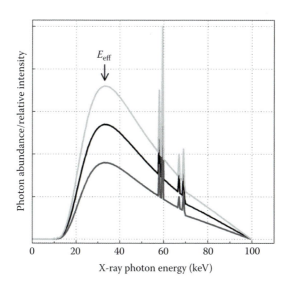

Figure 4.9 Variation of the intensity of the X-ray beam with mA. The graph shows that the only feature to change is the height (or size) of the curve and that change will represent a doubling of the area under the curve for a doubling of the mA.

- The maximum photon energy achievable will increase and so E-max will increase to match the higher keV applied across the tube.
- There will be an increase in the average energy of each photon of X-rays comprising the X-ray beam and therefore the peak energy (kVp) will shift towards a higher energy value (i.e. to the right along the energy axis). It also follows that if the peak energy of the X-ray beam is one-third to one-half of the maximum energy then as the E-max increases, the kVp must shift proportionately.
- There will be more opportunities for individual X-ray photons to be produced and therefore as the total number of photons increases, the intensity of the X-ray beam must increase.

All of these changes are represented in **Figure 4.10**.

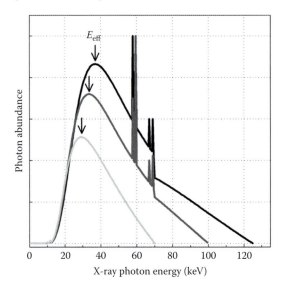

Figure 4.10 The change of the X-ray spectrum with applied kilovoltage.

Logic will tell you that each of the changes mentioned above will be reversed if there is a reduction in the applied tube voltage. We can therefore determine that:

- beam quality $\propto keV^2$;
- beam intensity $\propto keV$.

The impact of filtration on the X-ray beam

The X-ray beam, in the process of leaving the X-ray tube, will pass through certain components of the tube. These are collectively called 'inherent filtration':

- The glass or ceramic envelope which maintains the vacuum.
- The cooling oil.
- The window of the X-ray tube, which is usually made of beryllium due its low atomic number (which means it will not absorb too many of the X-rays).

Additionally, every X-ray tube you use will have external or added filtration added to preferentially remove the lower energy, 'softer'

X-rays from the beam. Usually these filters will be made of aluminium for use with the diagnostic range of X-ray energies. Aluminium is used because it has a low atomic number and will therefore be more likely to absorb (or scatter) low energy photons and more likely to leave higher energy (useful) photons to form the radiographic image.

The lower energy X-radiation would have sufficient energy to increase the radiation dose to the superficial tissues of the patient, but it would not be able to penetrate through the patient and contribute to the process of radiographic image formation (or tumour treatment in the case of a radiotherapy beam therefore only add to patient dose).

The amount of filtration added will depend on the maximum generating voltage of the tube (i.e. the maximum kV available to the radiographer), but it is usual to have between 1.5 and 2.5 mm.

In order that we can understand the impact of the X-ray beam on the patient, we must first understand what effect filtration will have on the beam and the best way to do that is to consider what happens when inherent filtration and added filtration is allowed to impact on the X-ray beam.

In **Figure 4.11**, you can see that the higher energy components of the beam remain broadly the same, however, the lower energy components will vary.

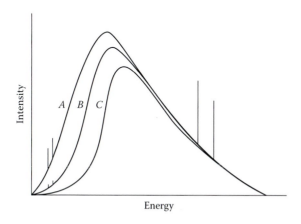

Figure 4.11 Continuous spectrum demonstrating the effect of filtration on effective energy.

- Spectrum A represents the beam without any filtration (i.e. it is still within the X-ray tube insert).
- Spectrum B represents the beam after it has passed through the envelope, the oil and the tube window (the inherent filtration) and it can be seen that some of the lower energy photons have been removed from the beam.
- Spectrum C represents the beam after it has passed through the added filtration at which point most of the lower energy, less useful X-ray photons have been removed.

The graph shows us that:

- The process of filtration will not affect E-max (because the higher energy photons are largely unaffected by the process of beam filtration).
- The intensity of the beam will be decreased as the beam passes through increasing thicknesses of the filter (due to the lower energy photons being absorbed or scattered).
- The average energy of the beam (represented by the position of the peak of the graph along the energy axis) will increase with additional thicknesses of filter material.

We can therefore determine that beam quality is proportional to filtration and beam intensity and is inversely proportional to filtration.

MCQs

1. **With reference to the interaction of electrons from the cathode with atoms of the anode, what percentage of heat typically occurs?**
   a. 1 per cent
   b. 10 per cent
   c. 2 per cent
   d. 99 per cent.

2. **The inner envelope of an X-ray tube is usually made from:**
   a. Ceramics
   b. Lead
   c. Copper
   d. Aluminium.

3. Typical anode angles in general diagnostic X-ray tubes (excluding mammography) tend to be between:
   a. 4 and 6°
   b. 16 and 20°
   c. 25 and 30°
   d. 30 and 45°.

4. The X-ray tube incorporates an angled target in order to:
   a. Decrease the size of real focal spot
   b. Decrease the size of apparent focal spot
   c. Increase the size of apparent focal spot
   d. Increase length of target track.

5. The following material is added to the anode disc of a rotating X-ray tube to prevent the crazing effect:
   a. Molybdenum
   b. Carbon
   c. Rhenium
   d. Copper.

6. Modern anode discs, which contain more than one material in their construction, may be referred to as a
   a. Bi-anode
   b. Double anode
   c. Compound anode
   d. Rare-earth anode.

7. The added filtration of a diagnostic X-ray tube typically consists of:
   a. Aluminium or copper
   b. Aluminium and beryllium
   c. Copper or tin
   d. Tin or lead.

8. The filtration of an X-ray beam has the effect of:
   a. Improving the quality of the transmitted X-ray beam
   b. Increasing the quantity of the transmitted X-ray beam
   c. Reducing the quantity and decreasing quality of the transmitted X-ray beam
   d. Improving the quality and increasing quantity of the transmitted X-ray beam.

9. **When X-rays are produced, the maximum energy of an X-ray photon is determined by the:**
   a. mA
   b. mAs
   c. Temperature of the filament
   d. keV.

10. **When X-rays are emitted from the X-ray tube, the minimum energy of the radiation beam is determined by the:**
    a. Added filtration
    b. mAs
    c. mA
    d. Exposure time.

CHAPTER 5
X-RAY INTERACTIONS IN MATTER

INTRODUCTION

The aim of this chapter is to give the practitioner an understanding of the interactions of X-rays with matter. It is important to understand the principles of attenuation processes and be able to adjust exposure and other factors to enhance the image and reduce scatter, or remove it before it affects the image.

Learning objectives

The student should be able to:
- Understand and explain the principles of attenuation.
- Understand and explain the processes of Compton scatter and the photoelectric effect.
- Explain the terms 'linear' and 'mass' attenuation coefficient and there significance to radiography.

INTERACTIONS OF X-RAYS IN MATTER

X-rays will interact with all manner of things both inside the X-ray tube and after they have left it, but as practitioners we are primarily interested in how they interact with patients and detectors, in terms of producing the image and managing the radiation dose to the patient.

The principles of interaction are similar for all materials and they are primarily affected by the atomic number of the medium and the energy of the X-rays themselves.

It is a simple fact that the interactions we are discussing occur between photons of X-rays and atoms (or to be more exact, the electrons contained within atoms) of the medium which is irradiated. If we want to reduce the number of interactions therefore, we must either reduce the number of photons in the beam or reduce the number of atoms exposed (or both). The use of tissue displacement bands (often called 'compression bands') will reduce the number of atoms in the beam and collimation of the beam will reduce both the number of photons released from the tube and the number of atoms irradiated.

All radiography practice should be based on an understanding of these basic facts; they are the very essence of radiation dose reduction.

It must be clearly understood that a patient will only receive a 'radiation dose' if energy from the X-ray beam is deposited in their tissues. If all photons were to go straight through tissues then radiography would be a process which was risk free in terms of radiation risk. However, it is probably clear to you that if all of the X-rays were to pass straight through tissues without any interaction there would be no radiographic image either!

Attenuation

In a clinical environment, all X-ray beams (although not all X-ray photons) will interact with the medium through which they pass and therefore, to a greater or lesser extent, the beam will be attenuated. To attenuate is to weaken or reduce something and in the case of the diagnostic X-ray beam, that reduction occurs through two processes: absorption or scattering of the photons.

It therefore follows that as a beam of radiation passes through a medium, any one of three things can happen to its photons (**Figure 5.1**). They can:
- Pass straight through the medium;
- Be absorbed by the medium and therefore cease to exist;
- Undergo scattering where, following the interaction event, the photon of radiation will travel in an entirely new and different direction.

It can be stated then that for all diagnostic X-ray beams: attenuation = absorption + scatter.

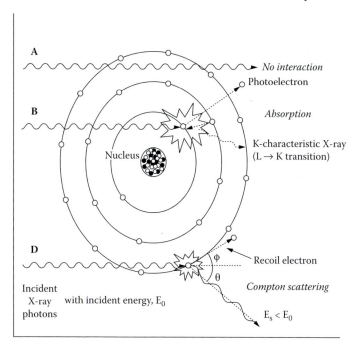

Figure 5.1 Summary of interactions.

Linear attenuation coefficient (µ)

The chances of any particular X-ray photon interacting with a given atom are not great at all, however, every time a patient undergoes an X-ray examination, so many millions of atoms are exposed to many X-ray photons that it is inevitable that some absorption and scattering events will take place.

An estimation of the probability of absorption and scattering events occurring in any given material can be gained by considering the linear attenuation coefficient (represented by µ (the Greek letter mu)) for that material.

A coefficient is simply a number or symbol which, in this case, represents the ability of a medium or material to attenuate radiation per unit thickness of the material (thickness being a linear measurement, hence the term 'linear attenuation coefficient').

In order to fully understand the mathematical concept of linear attenuation for X- and γ-radiation, it is necessary to study the exponential process and the role of linear attenuation within it. However, this book is intended to be a practical handbook and further background detail in this area is left to other authors.

It is probably sufficient to say here that:

The total linear attenuation coefficient (μ) is the fraction of X-rays removed from the beam per unit thickness of the irradiated medium.

The total linear attenuation coefficient represents the sum of all of the absorption and scattering events which occur during the passage of an X-ray beam through the material.

- τ (tau) is the symbol used to determine the linear *absorption* coefficient for the photoelectric absorption process and
- σ (sigma) is used to represent the linear *scattering* coefficient for Compton scatter.

Therefore, for diagnostic X-ray beams:

$$\mu = \tau + \sigma.$$

i.e. total attenuation = photoelectric absorption + Compton scatter.

The main problem with using linear attenuation coefficient as the guide to how much attenuation will occur in a given thickness of material is that as the physical conditions of the material change (a material could be a solid, a liquid or a gas), then the accuracy of that coefficient can change. If, for example, a material was heated and expanded, it is extremely likely that its thickness would change (i.e. its volume would increase, its density would decrease and the number of atoms per unit volume would decrease proportionately).

This would mean that the linear attenuation coefficient would also change. However, if the linear attenuation coefficient were divided by the density of the medium, the numerical value would remain proportionally consistent. In this context, density is represented by ρ (the Greek letter rho): (total) mass attenuation coefficient (μ/ρ).

The mass attenuation coefficient is, therefore, the linear attenuation coefficient (represented by μ) divided by the density of the medium (represented by ρ) and this ratio removes the anomalies caused by any physical changes which may occur as a result of environmental conditions.

The mass attenuation coefficient is therefore a more reliable measure of attenuation under a variety of circumstances and will be referred to during the remainder of this section.

Total mass attenuation coefficient can be defined as:

The fractional reduction of X-rays per unit mass of the medium.

It will comprise the individual mass absorption and scattering coefficients: τ/ρ is the mass absorption coefficient (for the photoelectric process) and σ/ρ is the mass scattering coefficient (for Compton scatter).

Therefore for diagnostic X-ray beams:

$$\frac{\mu}{\rho} = \frac{\tau}{\rho} + \frac{\sigma}{\rho}.$$

i.e. total mass attenuation = mass absorption + mass scattering.

THE PROCESSES OF ATTENUATION IN DIAGNOSTIC RADIOGRAPHY

Attenuation coefficients can help us to understand how much attenuation will occur based on a given set of circumstances, but we also need to understand how the individual processes occur. The remainder of this chapter will consider the attenuation processes which contribute to the radiographic image. Consideration will be given to the impact of the processes on image formation and on patient radiation doses.

Just to remind you:

attenuation = absorption + scatter.

There are four processes of attenuation which need to be mentioned but, from a diagnostic perspective, only two of these need to be described and thoroughly understood. The four processes are:

1. Elastic (unmodified) scatter
2. Pair production

3. Photoelectric absorption
4. Compton (inelastic or modified) scatter.

Elastic scatter

Elastic scatter occurs between low energy photons and electrons which are bound into atoms of the target material. This process has little significance in diagnostic imaging, largely because many of the low energy photons have been removed from the beam prior to reaching the patient.

Pair production

This process does not occur in diagnostic X-ray beams. The process only occurs with a photon energy of 1.02 MeV and above. The photon interacts with the nucleus of an atom and produces a positron and an electron. Positron annihilation is the basis of positron emission tomography (PET) scanning.

Photoelectric absorption

The previous processes are not really relevant to diagnostic radiography, however, the photoelectric process described here is very relevant because it occurs predominantly in the X-ray energy range used in diagnostic radiography. The photoelectric effect is the main source of the data for digital image production in diagnostic radiography.

This process can be best described by annotating **Figure 5.2**:

1. The incoming photon must have an energy which is equal to or slightly greater than the binding (ionisation) energy of the electron. (As the beam energy increases the process is much less likely to occur.)
2. The bound electron will be ejected from the atom leaving it ionised. Any excess energy over and above the binding energy used by the photon to remove the electron is donated to the electron as kinetic energy and therefore the photon has donated all of its energy and ceases to exist (i.e. its energy has been absorbed). The electron will travel through the material until the donated kinetic energy has been used, when it comes to rest and acts like any other electron.

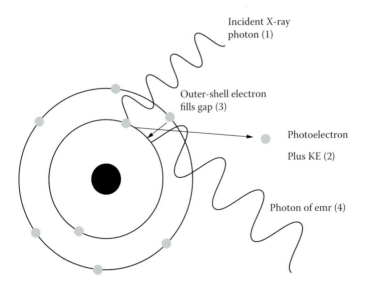

Figure 5.2 Photoelectric effect.

3. The vacancy in the electron shell occurring as a result of the ionisation process in (2) will be filled by an electron from a shell further away from the nucleus of the atom.
4. A photon of electromagnetic radiation will be released as a result of the electron transition in (3) above. The energy of this photon will be dependent entirely on the atomic number of the material (as it is the attractive force of the nucleus due to the number of protons it contains which directly determines the binding energy of the electrons in each electron orbital or shell). If this process occurs in patient tissues, the energy of the transition photon will be very low and it is likely that it will fall in the infrared part of the electromagnetic spectrum as heat.

This interaction process will therefore see the X-ray energy carried in some of the incoming photons absorbed by human tissue with the associated potential for cellular and chromosomal damage.

Photoelectric absorption coefficients

The mass attenuation coefficient (which, in this process, is effectively an absorption coefficient as there is no scatter involved) for the photoelectric process is dependent on two factors:

1. The atomic number of the medium (Z), and
2. The energy of the X-ray beam (E).

In broad terms, we find that:

$$\frac{\tau}{\rho} \propto Z^3.$$

- This means that relatively small changes in the atomic number of the medium give rise to reasonably significant changes in the absorption of X-rays.
- Many radiographic examinations (including all extremity examinations) rely on the ability of the radiographer to distinguish between bone and soft tissues.
- As an estimation, it can be assumed that soft tissue has an atomic number of 7.4, while the atomic number of bone is around 13.
- Therefore, if those numbers are both cubed (as per the formula above) we can see that rather than bone absorbing slightly more X-rays than soft tissue, it actually absorbs more than five times as much.
- This will have a significant impact on the level of image contrast between bone and soft tissue that we see when viewing extremity images, for example, and it will improve our ability to make bony diagnoses from plain radiographic images.
- The process is also put to good use in mammographic imaging where a primary aim is to demonstrate 'microcalcifications' (often the first sign of breast tumours) against the soft tissue background of the otherwise normal breast.

Additionally, we find that:

$$\frac{\tau}{\rho} \propto \frac{1}{E^3}.$$

- Essentially, this means that the chance of the photoelectric process occurring decreases very rapidly as the radiation beam energy increases.
- It is therefore clear that if we wish to utilize the photoelectric effect to enhance image contrast, then we shall need to ensure that relatively low beam energies are used. It is no coincidence that much of our work as diagnostic radiographers is undertaken in the 60–150 kV range as that is where the photoelectric absorption process predominates when soft tissues and bone are being X-rayed.
- We would tend to use the upper part of this kV bracket when a greater degree of beam penetration is required, e.g. for a thicker patient body part, but in extremity work for example, the tendency is to use an image-enhancing lower kV of around 60.
- The downside to this practice is that by using lower beam energies to enhance the probability of the photoelectric process occurring, we are also increasing the amount of energy absorption and therefore increasing the dose to the patient.
- It does, however, affirm the point that, after the need for a radiographic examination has been determined, the production of a high quality image becomes the priority to fully justify the inevitable (if often small) radiation dose. If the two equations above are combined, then we can see clearly that there are two major influences on the ability to utilize the photoelectric effect: one which can be controlled by the radiographer (the beam energy) and one which cannot (the atomic composition of the patient).

$$\frac{\tau}{\rho} \propto \frac{Z^3}{E^3}.$$

- The graph in **Figure 5.3** confirms the point that the probability of the photoelectric absorption process decreases sharply with increasing energy, however, it also appears to show a couple of anomalies where the probability spikes at certain energies.
- This happens because each electron orbital has a different binding energy for its electrons depending on how far that orbital is from the nucleus.

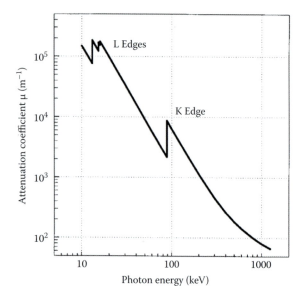

Figure 5.3 Graph to show a representative mass absorption coefficient (τ/ρ) in human soft tissue.

- The graph shows the probability of the photoelectric process decreasing inversely with respect to the beam energy, however, at a certain energy (depending on the nature of the atom) the binding or ionisation energy of the electrons in the next orbital of the atom will be reached.
- Up to that point, the electrons in that orbital could not be involved in the process, but as soon as that binding energy value is achieved, additional electrons can be involved and as the photoelectric process occurs as a result of a photon of X-ray energy interacting with an electron, whenever additional electrons become available, the probability of the process occurring must increase.
- Hence, there is a sharp upward spike in the graph at the exact binding energy of the electrons in the next orbital and then the probability immediately begins to fall away again as the beam energy continues to increase.

■ A further spike may be achieved, but if we assume that this corresponds to the inclusion of the K-orbital electrons being involved, then there will be no additional spikes as the K-orbital is the innermost orbital (and its electrons have the highest binding energy of any in that atom) and so the probability line for that process in that atom falls away towards zero.

We now need to consider what will happen if the incoming photon has an energy which is not equal to or slightly greater than the binding energy of the bound electrons (as was the case with the photoelectric absorption process), but has one which is much greater.

Compton scatter

This process will meet the parameters set out in the last paragraph above. It occurs when the energy of the incoming photon is considerably greater than the binding energy of the electron involved. In the case of the Compton scattering process, the photon energy is so much greater than the electron binding energy that some texts describe the electron as being a 'free' electron. This somewhat confusing term can lead you to think that the electron is not bound into an atom at all. This is not the case, it is a term which is used to try and indicate the mega-mismatch between the two energies involved i.e. the X-ray photon and the weekly-bound electron.

Once again, we will use annotations in **Figure 5.4** to explain the process which leads to the production of Compton scatter.

1. An incoming photon with an energy much in excess of the binding energy of the electron, interacts with and ejects the electron from the atom.

2. The ejected electron will receive a proportion of the photon's energy as kinetic energy and, as with the photoelectric process, will go on to interact with other atoms until all of its energy has been dispersed. This deposition of energy into tissues clearly means that there is some absorption of radiation energy and that the patient receives a small radiation dose as a result of this process occurring.

3. The photon undergoes a change in direction as a direct result of the collision with the electron and is therefore scattered. It also experiences a reduction in energy which is equivalent to the binding energy of the electron and the kinetic energy acquired by it as it left the atom.

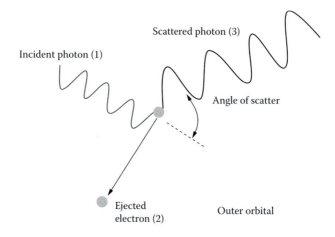

Figure 5.4 Compton scatter.

- The angle of scatter can be directly associated with the energy lost by the photon and is greatest when the photon is backscattered along its original path (i.e. it is scattered through 180°).
- The angle of scattering is greatest at lower photon energies and smallest at higher energies. As the beam energy increases, there is a reduction in the amount of energy donated to the electron and therefore the overall amount of scatter is reduced.
- This may be a difficult concept to understand as you are likely to be aware that anti-scatter grids tend to be used for thicker patient parts and with higher kVs.
- However, what must be remembered is that although there will be an overall reduction in the amount of scatter at higher beam energies, it is also the case that more of that scatter will be travelling at a reduced scattering angle (i.e. in a forward direction, towards the image receptor); therefore, the anti-scatter grid is more likely to be needed at these higher energies.

Compton scatter coefficients

- The mass attenuation coefficient (which, in this process, is effectively a scatter coefficient) for the Compton scatter process is dependent on two factors: (1) the energy of the beam and (2) the electron density of the medium.
- For this process, we find that:

$$\frac{\sigma}{\rho} \propto \frac{1}{E} .$$

- This reflects the statement above indicating that as the energy of the beam increases, so the probability of Compton scatter occurring is reduced. The probability of the Compton scattering process occurring is also seen to be directly proportional to the electron density of the attenuator:

$$\sigma/\rho - \propto \text{ electron density}$$

  The electron density of a material represents the number of electrons per unit mass of the medium.
- As you will know from your study of atomic structure, the great majority of the mass is found in the nucleus of the atom with each proton and neutron accounting for approximately one atomic mass unit each.
- In most atoms, there will normally be an equal number of protons and electrons (to maintain the electrical balance).
- It therefore follows that all atoms with equal numbers of protons and neutrons (which accounts for virtually all atoms at the lower end of the periodic table), will have a mass:electron ratio of 2:1.
- Further up the periodic table (where atoms have a tendency to become more unstable), we find that the ratio is closer to 2.5:1, as there are more neutrons than protons.
- However, there is one atom which is different in this context because there is just one that does not have any neutrons at all.
- Hydrogen, as you will recall, has only one nucleon (a proton) in its nucleus and therefore it has an atomic mass of 1. It also

has one electron and so it follows that the mass: electron ratio (electron density) for hydrogen is 1:1.

- This means that hydrogen has an electron density which is at least twice as great as any other atom.
- As stated above, the probability of Compton scatter occurring is proportional to the electron density of the material and therefore any medium which contains large amounts of hydrogen will produce greater amounts of Compton scatter.
- Probably the most commonly encountered material with a high hydrogen content will be water, with two hydrogen atoms out of a total of three atoms per molecule.
- In clinical radiography, the materials we consider to have a high water content are soft tissues and fat and it follows therefore, that the largest amounts of Compton scatter will be encountered anywhere where there are significant amounts of these materials. As radiographers, you should think about the X-ray examinations and patient types where secondary radiation grids are needed – these are probably areas with larger amounts of soft tissue present.
- Don't forget, you are likely to be able to remove large amounts of soft tissue (including fatty tissues) from the image by using displacement bands which will really reduce the amount of scatter produced. This is an effective and much underused dose reduction measure.

MCQs

1. **In diagnostic radiography, photoelectric absorption occurs most in:**
   a. Air
   b. Bone
   c. Tissue
   d. Fat.

2. **Attenuation of an X-ray beam within matter is not affected by:**
   a. Compton scatter
   b. Photoelectric absorption
   c. Transmission of X-rays
   d. Atomic number and electron density.

3. **Mass attenuation increases with:**
   a. Decreasing mass number
   b. Increasing temperature of the material
   c. Increasing beam energy
   d. Electron density.

4. **The linear attenuation coefficient:**
   a. Defines the probability of absorption or scattering process taking place
   b. Is higher for fat than soft tissue for the same photon energy
   c. Decreases attenuation per cm of the attenuating medium
   d. Defines the fractional reduction in X-rays per unit mass of the attenuator.

5. **Which interaction process does not take place in the range of intensities of a diagnostic beam?**
   a. Compton scatter
   b. Photoelectric absorption
   c. Pair production
   d. Coherent scatter.

6. **The probability of photoelectric absorption occurring is greatest when:**
   a. The energy of the incoming photon is equal to or just above the ionisation energy of the atom with which it is interacting.
   b. The energy of the incoming photon is much greater than the ionisation energy of the atom with which it is interacting.
   c. The energy of the incoming photon is less than the ionisation energy of the atom with which it is interacting.
   d. The energy of the incoming photon is much less than the ionisation energy of the atom with which it is interacting.

7. **As the photon energy of an X-ray beam increases:**
   a. The incidence of Compton scattering increases.
   b. The incidence of photoelectric absorption increases.
   c. The incidence of Compton scattering and photoelectric absorption both decrease.
   d. The incidence of Compton scattering increases and photoelectric absorption decreases.

8. **The mass attenuation coefficient is:**
   a. Equal to the linear attenuation process multiplied by the density
   b. Equal to the linear attenuation process divided by the density
   c. Independent of atomic number
   d. Different for ice and water.

9. **The probability of a Compton interaction is:**
   a. Proportional to electron density of the medium
   b. Inversely proportional to electron density
   c. Proportional to atomic number
   d. Proportional to the beam energy.

10. **In the photoelectric absorption process:**
   a. All energy of the photon is passed to the free electron.
   b. No ionisation of the atom takes place.
   c. The vacancy from the photoelectron is filled from an inner shell electron.
   d. The vacancy from the photoelectron is filled by an electron from an orbital (shell) further out in the atom.

CHAPTER 6

PRINCIPLES OF RADIATION DETECTION AND IMAGE FORMATION

INTRODUCTION

The aim of this chapter is to explore how radiation is detected, measured, quantified and used in order to produce images.

There are various types of radiation detector which are designed for different purposes within medical imaging. There are automatic exposure devices and computed tomography (CT) detectors, as well as those used within general radiographic and fluoroscopic imaging.

This chapter will begin by looking generally at the types of detector we may come across in the radiography department, but the focus and bias later in the chapter revolves specifically around large field detectors used in general radiography.

Learning objectives

The students should be able to:

- Discuss how radiation is detected, measured, quantified and used in order to control exposure, as well as produce images.
- Discuss various detectors and how they are used for different clinical purposes.
- Discuss the benefits and limitations of various detector types used within different imaging systems.

DESIRABLE CHARACTERISTICS OF RADIATION DETECTORS

There are a number of characteristics which are considered for any kind of radiation detector. The main ones include:

- **Absorption efficiency** is clearly desirable that a detector is able to absorb as many of the incident X-rays as possible. The overall absorption is dependent on the physical density (atomic number, size, thickness).
- **Conversion efficiency** is essentially the ability of a detector to convert absorbed X-ray energy into a usable electronic signal.
- **Capture efficiency** is dependent on the physical area of the face plate minus the interspace between individual detectors and side and end walls.
- **Dose efficiency** is influenced by both conversion and capture efficiency. Typical dose efficiency is anywhere between 50 and 80 per cent for individual detector designs, but nearer 30–60 per cent for flat panel detectors.
- **Temporal response** should be as fast as possible and is the time it takes the detector to absorb the radiation, send a signal and prepare for the next reading.
- **Phosphorescence or afterglow** affects temporal response; until the detector has stopped giving off a signal, it cannot detect another signal.
- **Wide dynamic range,** in its simplest terms, is the range of radiation intensities the detectors are sensitive to.
- **High reproducibility and stability** help avoid drift and resultant detector fluctuation or noise variation.

DETECTIVE QUANTUM EFFICIENCY

Detective quantum efficiency (DQE) is often a measure that is quoted in order to make comparisons between various imaging systems and takes account of all the characteristics mentioned above.

The DQE describes how well an imaging system performs, essentially based on its overall signal-to-noise ratio (SNR) when compared against a theoretical ideal detector. It is essentially a measure of how much of the available signal is degraded by the imaging system.

A very simplistic way of looking at it is that the DQE value represents the probability of a signal being produced by the detector system. A DQE of 50 per cent means that approximately 50 per cent of the available quanta is used by the system (compared to an ideal system) to produce a signal.

If we consider two imaging systems with different DQEs, but the same SNR, the one with the higher DQE would require less signal and consequently less radiation exposure for the same eventual image quality. So, in some ways, it can almost be used as a measure of dose efficiency.

The actual measures of true DQEs are a little more complex as DQE is also affected by spatial frequency. The DQE of a particular system can also vary as signal values change; the signal is effectively produced by the exposure (especially the kV value), as well as the detector's internal structure. The same system will probably have a slightly different DQE for different kV values. As such, manufacturers often supply a series of graphs of DQE plotted against spatial frequency and kV.

Figure 6.1 illustrates the complex relationships involved in assessing DQE. The main reason it is often quoted is that it is a helpful measure of detector performance but, if taken at face value, can mislead without careful consideration of how it is derived.

Ionisation chambers

In their simplest configuration, ionisation chambers consist of a positive (anode) and a negative (cathode) electrode plate which are placed at opposite ends of a sealed chamber (**Figure 6.2**). The material used to construct the chamber is an electrical insulator. The space in between the electrodes forms the sensitive volume and this is filled with a gas, such as air.

The electrodes are supplied with a voltage, but as the chamber is made of an insulating material and the air in between the electrode plates is also naturally a good insulator; then a current will not flow between the electrodes.

However, when X-rays pass through the chamber, some of them interact with the outer shell electrons of the atoms that make up air

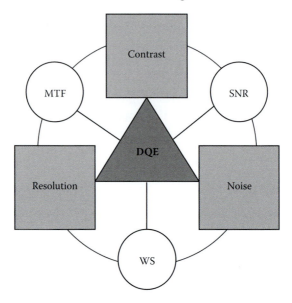

Figure 6.1 Factors affecting the DQE: Modulation transfer function (MTF) takes account of the combined effects of resolution and contrast and how they influence each other; signal-to-noise ratio (SNR) takes account of the combined effects of contrast and noise and how they influence each other; Weiner spectra (WS) is essentially the combined effects of noise and resolution and how they influence each other (see Lança and Silva, 2009).

inside the chamber. This causes the ejection of the electron from its orbit. This results in a free negatively charged electron (negative ion) and a positively charged ion. This process is known as 'ionisation'.

The negative ions flow to the positive electrode and the positive ions flow to the negative electrode. This causes a current to flow between the positive and negative electrode plates. The electrons move much faster as they have much less mass than the positive ions so the charge is usually measured from the anode.

The amount of current that flows is directly related to how much of the air is ionised, which in turn, is dependent on the amount of radiation passing through the sensitive volume.

Air ionisation chambers are not used in clinical practice to form images due to their relatively large size, but they were widely used by

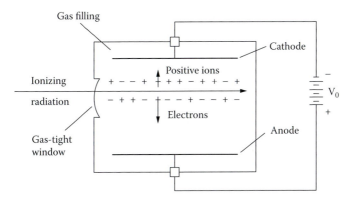

Figure 6.2 Ionisation chamber.

engineers to calibrate other radiation detectors in clinical departments. They are still used by standards laboratories to provide reference values against which all other detectors are measured.

They do have an important clinical role to play and that is in automatic exposure control (AEC) circuits which exploit the desirable characteristics of this type of detector.

IONISATION CHAMBERS USED FOR AUTOMATIC EXPOSURE CONTROL CIRCUITS

The sensitive volume can be made very thin allowing it to be positioned between the patient and image receptor and is constructed of radiolucent materials so it is not visible on the resultant image.

The X-rays emerging from the patient pass through the automatic exposure control (AEC) on to the imaging system (**Figure 6.3**). As the detector is very thin and contains gas, relatively few interactions take place so only a tiny amount of the primary beam is absorbed, but it is enough to cause ionisation within the detector and produce a small signal in proportion to the X-ray energy passing through it.

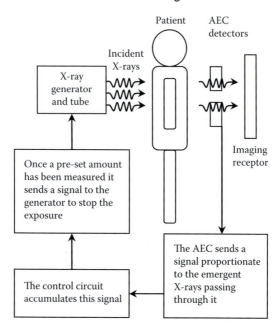

Figure 6.3 Demonstrates the set up for an automatic exposure control (AEC).

The circuitry is preprogrammed to measure the size of this signal and once it reaches a predetermined level terminate the exposure.

The chambers are typically around 5 or 6 cm long by 3–4 cm wide but only a few millimetres deep. The device is crude in some respects as it is influenced by all the incident radiation that passes through its area. In other words, it cannot take account of variations in X-ray intensity within its 6 × 4 cm dimensions; it simply measures the total amount passing through that area. As such, it is important that the radiographer takes into account the patient's anatomy that overlies the AEC area.

In general radiography, we use a system of three or five chambers: Correct exposure can only be achieved if we select an appropriate chamber for the anatomy overlying it or we deliberately increase or decrease the sensitivity of the chamber to account for an area we know will result in an over good collimation is essential when using AEC's to reduce scatter in an over- or underexposed image. **Figure 6.4** indicates where the AEC chambers may be positioned on an abdominal X-ray with 3 chambers.

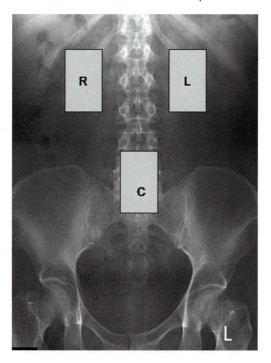

Figure 6.4 Position of the automatic exposure control (AEC) chambers on an abdominal X-ray, where R is right AEC; L, left AEC; C, central AEC.

Xenon gas detectors

Xenon gas detectors are a form of ionisation chamber and these were common on premultislice CT scanners (**Figure 6.5**).

Thin tungsten plates separate the chambers and also act as electrodes with a large potential difference applied between plates. Positive electrodes are interspaced with negative electrodes as in **Figure 6.5**.

As with individual air ionization chambers, once emergent X-rays enter the sensitive volume it causes ionization which allows current to flow between the electrodes creating a signal. However, the objective here is different to the ionisation chambers used in AECs that only interfere very slightly with the X-rays passing through the volume so that the vast majority of radiation is not absorbed. The detectors in

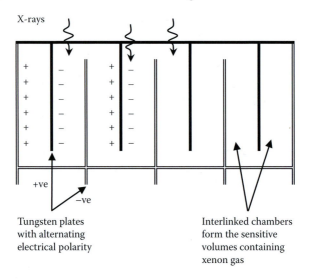

X-rays

+ve

−ve

Tungsten plates
with alternating
electrical polarity

Interlinked chambers
form the sensitive
volumes containing
xenon gas

Figure 6.5 Xenon gas detector.

xenon systems are used instead to form the image. As such, they are designed to absorb as much of the emergent radiation as possible.

As with air, the atoms of xenon gas are much further apart than liquids or solids, so they naturally have very low absorption efficiency. The amount of space within a CT scanner gantry is limited, so it is not feasible to use large chambers in order to obtain reasonable absorption efficiency, so manufacturers employed two methods to increase the poor natural absorption efficiency. The first step was to increase the length of the chambers. The second was to increase the density of atoms per unit volume by squeezing more into the sensitive volume. This is achieved by pressurizing the sensitive volume typically to anywhere from 10 and 30 atmospheres; xenon is used as the gas of choice, as it is very stable even under pressure. Both the steps described above significantly increase the chance of interactions between the X-rays and atoms of xenon gas thereby significantly increasing the absorption efficiency and therefore the sensitivity of this type of detector, allowing much smaller detectors to be used.

The downside of this design is that the chamber itself has to have relatively thick walls, including the face plate, to withstand the pressure, resulting in some of the radiation being absorbed before it hits the sensitive volume. Even so, these detectors have zero afterglow and exceptional temporal response which are very desirable characteristics.

As they have exceptional afterglow and temporal response properties, they are excellent in applications where fast switching is required, such as CT. They can detect X-rays and send a signal in a fraction of the time it takes other types of detectors to respond.

If many detectors are added together with the same sensitive volume dimensions, the individual chambers can be interlinked so that the gas is free to move throughout the whole array. This means the chambers all have identical pressures and all the individual sensitive volumes will respond almost identically to a certain amount of radiation requiring very little calibration in comparison to other detector designs.

Scintillation crystals/photocathode multiplier

Scintillation crystals/photocathode multipliers have a role as scintillation counters within nuclear medicine and the gamma camera is an extensively modified scintillation counter (**Figure 6.6**). They were also used as an early type of detector primarily with first and second generation CT scanners.

X-ray and gamma radiation detection is essentially a three-stage process:

1. A solid scintillation crystal captures and converts X-rays into light.

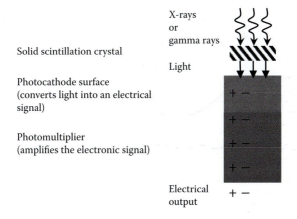

Figure 6.6 Scintillation crystal and photocathode arrangement.

91

2. Light is then converted into a small electrical signal by the photocathode.

3. Finally, a photomultiplier is used to amplify the signal into a much larger useful electronic signal.

This type of detector is used in medical imaging but no longer to produce images from X-ray systems. It was notorious for drifting and afterglow, resulting in image degradation and inaccuracies.

Scintillation crystal/photocathode X-ray image intensifier

One technology that is very similar and is still being used clinically is the X-ray image intensifier (**Figure 6.7**). It only merits a brief description as this technology is slowly being phased out of production.

Image production is a four-stage process with the whole system encased in a vacuum tube:

1. A solid scintillation crystal coats the inside of the vacuum tube face plate. It captures and converts X-rays into light.

2. Light is then converted into a small photoelectrical signal by the photocathode.

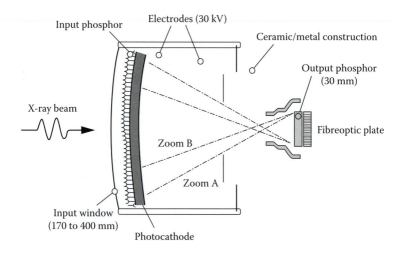

Figure 6.7 Image intensifier.

3. The photoelectrical signal is accelerated and focused by high kV electrodes arranged around the inside diameter of the tube. The electrodes decreasing in circumference along the length of the tube towards the output phosphor.

4. The highly focused and energetic photoelectric signal strikes the output phosphor which subsequently converts the signal to light.

The light output can then be recorded using a video camera. Older analogue systems used either vidicon or plumbicon video cameras. More modern equipment uses a solid-state charged couple device (CCD)-based camera. The diagram above shows optical fibres connecting the output phosphor to the CCD system which will be digitised. This technology is currently the most prevalent form of digital fluoroscopy in clinical use, but its days are numbered and it will slowly be phased out of clinical use.

Scintillation crystals/silicon photodiode multiplier

Solid-state type of detectors (**Figure 6.8**) are used extensively within CT scanners, but the reason they are included in this book is that their principles of operation are also very similar to some of the large field detectors that are discussed as the next topic.

The latest solid crystal detector materials have many advantages over their predecessors, including high stability and relatively small size, together with possible cost savings.

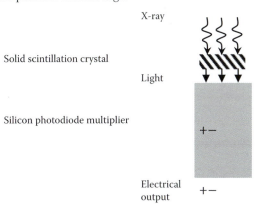

Figure 6.8 Solid state detector.

Radiation detection is essentially a two-stage process this time:

1. A solid scintillation crystal captures and converts X-rays into light.
2. The light is then converted into a useable electrical signal by the photodiode. The signal is proportional to the quantity and quality of the incident X-rays.

The latest solid-state detectors of this type have virtually zero afterglow and are used almost exclusively in spiral scanners, certainly the case for multislice/spiral scanners and those capable of CT fluoroscopy.

LARGE FIELD DETECTORS (OVERVIEW)

Large field detectors (LFDs) are detectors specifically designed to produce full-size radiographic images and replace film screen technology.

In order to produce an image, we need to detect the radiation that emerges from the patient's body being examined. Traditionally, this was performed using photographic emulsions which were either directly exposed to the emergent radiation or more commonly the emergent radiation was used to excite intensifying screen phosphors which caused them to produce light. This in turn was then used to produce a latent image in the photographic film emulsion that was subsequently processed using photographic chemicals.

The discrete individual detectors just mentioned would be simply too big physically to replace film screen technology, recording unacceptably large pixel sizes for general radiography. For example, modern multislice CT detectors are about as small as it gets in terms of the size of individual detectors, with the smallest currently available individual solid-state detectors being around 0.25 mm^2 across the face plate.

Even if we could get the detectors into an imaging plate thin enough to fit inside the bucky trays of conventional X-ray equipment, 0.25 mm^2 would only equate to two line pairs per millimetre (as a line pair is one black line and one white line). This is because we could only squeeze in four detectors in the x-axis by four detectors in the y-axis giving a total detector density of 16 detectors per mm^2.

The information or data measured by each detector is used to form the picture elements (pixels) in the resultant image, so this system would also give a pixel density of 16 pixels per mm². In reality, it would be even less than this when we account for the interspace material required to separate the individual detectors.

In order to get close to the resolution available with photographic emulsions, we need to use detector technology in a slightly different way.

A typical resolution of an older fast film screen technology used for larger body areas, such as the spine or abdomen, would be around five line pairs per millimetre. This is equivalent to a resultant image having ten pixels in each axis giving a pixel density of 100 pixels/mm², which also equates to a pixel resolution of 100 μm.

A traditional fine or detailed film screen combination used to image extremities would have to have an even greater resolution of at least ten line pairs per mm resulting in the equivalent of a pixel density of 400 pixels/mm², which equates to a pixel resolution of 50 μm.

In order to achieve these resolution values, then any digital detector system needs to have at least 400 individual areas per mm².

In radiography, rather than using individual detectors as we would with say CT, we use a large flat panel detector which produces a signal covering the whole area of the panel. We then need to put this into a grid known as the image matrix to make sense of it and this is where technology varies.

There are several manufacturers employing different technologies to detect/capture emergent radiation and subsequently produce an image. There are a few terms used when discussing these technologies, but the main categorisations are usually indirect and direct systems.

INDIRECT, DIRECT, COMPUTED AND DIGITAL RADIOGRAPHY

Indirect systems may either be computed radiography (CR) or indirect digital radiography (IDR), but in both cases X-rays are first absorbed and converted into light before being converted to an electrical signal.

Direct digital radiography (DDR) does not use an intermediate stage. The emergent X-rays directly cause the system to produce an electrical signal with no intermediate conversion of X-rays to light.

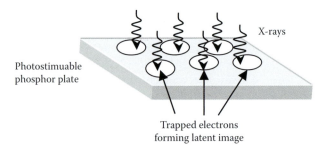

Photostimuable
phosphor plate

X-rays

Trapped electrons
forming latent image

Figure 6.9 Trapped electrons in a photostimuable phosphor (PSP) plate.

Computed radiography in detail

CR is a system that produces digital radiographic images utilizing imaging plates. From a user's perspective, it is very similar to film screen technology and was introduced because it does not generally require modifications to the X-ray equipment itself.

Following an exposure, the CR imaging plate retains a latent image in a similar way to previous film screen technology.

The differences occur when we process the latent image. Rather than being processed chemically, the latent CR image is scanned using a laser beam and digitised in a CR reader. The data are then sent to a computer for display, manipulation and archive.

Computed radiography using imaging plates (photostimuable phosphors (PSP)) is currently the most common imaging system (**Figure 6.9**).

CR plate construction

The imaging plates of CR systems are actually very similar to X-ray intensifier screens used in film screen technology in that their function is to absorb X-rays and convert them to light (**Figure 6.10**).

The main difference is that the phosphor material allows a delay to occur as part of the process which will be discussed in more detail shortly, but first we will look at the structure of the imaging plate itself.

There are some alternatives, but for our purposes we will use the principles associated with a PSP, such as barium fluoro-halide activated or doped by europium (Ba F Br$_x$ I$_{1-x}$:Eu).

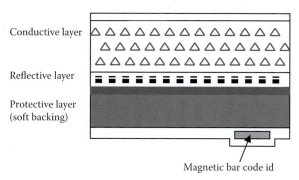

Figure 6.10 A cross-sectional representation of a computer radiography (CR) imaging plate. Please note the reflective layer is missing on a higher resolution version.

Production of the latent image

The emerging from the patient X-rays pass through the surface of the cassette on to the PSP. The X-rays interact with the electrons of the atoms within the PSP's conductive layer and transfer some energy. This causes the energised electrons of the PSP to move to a higher energy band within the atom's structure through the process of excitation (**Figure 6.11**).

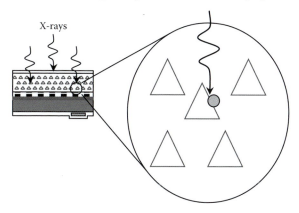

Figure 6.11 The triangles represent the crystalline structure of the photo-stimuable phosphor (PSP). The dot represents atoms within the crystalline structure that contain electrons in higher energy bands due to them capturing the energy from the X-ray beam.

The phosphor crystals are 'activated or doped' and this forms electron traps that hold on to the energised electron in this higher energy band. This forms the latent image as an analogue impression across the surface of the imaging plate. The plate will retain this impression until it is processed by the CR reader.

Processing or reading the latent CR impression

The energised electrons require additional energy in order to escape this energy band and return to their original/natural energy band. Refer to Chapter 3, for a further explanation of band theory.

The CR reader does this using a laser, with the light being the energy source. This gives the energised electrons enough extra energy to escape the trap. These electrons then fall back to their original energy band/orbit and, as they fall, they give off the excess energy in the form of different coloured light to that of the laser, usually blue light. This is measured by a moving scanning blue light detector (**Figure 6.12**).

The scanning detector measures light output in both the x- and y-axis. It does this by moving across the width of the imaging plate

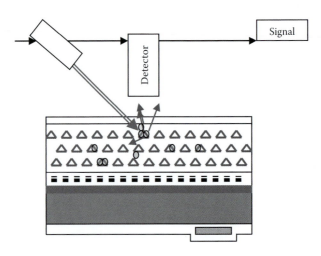

Figure 6.12 A diagram illustrating the construction of a computer radiography (CR) imaging plate being read.

while at the same time, the imaging plate passes through the reader (**Figure 6.13**).

Electronics track the x and y co-ordinates of the laser and detector as well as the quantity of light emitted at each point. The reader eventually builds up a map of the light output across the whole of the imaging plate in the form of a grid which becomes the image matrix. The data for individual squares within the grid form the picture elements or pixels in the final image. The data are sent to a computer workstation for display, manipulation and storage.

The rate at which the laser, detector and plate move through the reader can be slowed down allowing a greater number of measurements to be taken per mm^2 and this subsequently results in a finer matrix being formed. Typical CR resolutions range from 100 to 200 µm, so spatial resolution is lower than fine or detailed film screen technology. Fortunately, it benefits as from higher contrast resolution so is similar and generally regarded equivalent in terms of overall image quality.

The latest systems can employ multiple parallel lasers and light detectors/scanners which has significantly reduced the time it takes to read an imaging plate to under 10 seconds, which is a similar time to digital radiography (DR) technology.

Another criticism relates to processing of the imaging plates during mobile and theatre cases or other areas that did not have CR readers

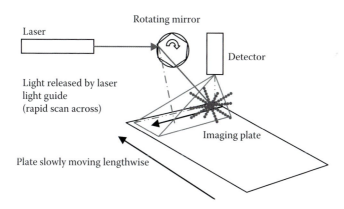

Figure 6.13 A simplistic diagram illustrating the main principles surrounding the reading of a photostimuable phosphor (PSP).

available nearby. This has been overcome lately with portable imaging plate readers being incorporated into mobile X-ray equipment or positioned around the hospital. The mobile CR readers can either be directly plugged into a wired network or even sent wirelessly to the main system.

Criticism of early systems was that they required relatively high exposures when compared to DR and fast film screen technology. Some manufacturers put two PSP layers one on either side of a transparent substrate to form the imaging plate, while others incorporated reflective layers. The result is a near doubling of sensitivity and lower noise, allowing almost a halving of exposure and subsequent dose to the patient. However, these techniques also cause spatial resolution (detail) to reduced.

Modern CR systems are at a point where processing times are within a few seconds of DR. Exposures and system sensitivity and therefore dose is very similar. They tend to be more compact and easier to use in challenging examinations and with the introduction of mobile readers, similar benefits are enjoyed away from the main imaging department.

Indirect digital radiography technology in detail

When the scintillator is exposed to X-rays, it immediately produces fluorescent light in proportion to the quantity and quality of X-rays interacting with it. The X-rays give electrons enough energy to move to a higher orbit, but unlike the phosphors used with CR, there are no electron traps so the energized electrons fall immediately back to their natural orbit releasing their excess energy as light. There are two main systems that come into this category: (1) those based on thin film transistor (TFT) technology and those based on charged coupled device (CCD) technology. Both designs use phosphors/scintillators that produce light when exposed to X-radiation. The differences in the systems revolve around how this light is detected and converted into a useful electrical signal that represents the quantity and quality of X-rays that fell on a particular area of the scintillator.

There are a few phosphors/scintillators that may be used by manufacturers, such as gadolinium oxisulphide (Gd_2O_2S) or caesium iodide (CsI). There are advantages and disadvantages with any scintillator, but generally speaking the materials are subclassified as being either structured or non-structured.

Non-structured scintillator crystals, such as Gd_2O_2S, are arranged randomly throughout the scintillator. The crystals themselves have similar dimensions in all planes, i.e. the face plate may be no larger or smaller than one of the side or oblique walls. Although not always the case, they tend to have a relatively high light output or conversion efficiency as the face plate is similar in dimension to any other surface of the crystal and there is, therefore, a relatively high chance of interaction with the X-ray beam in comparison to a structured crystal with a relatively small face plate.

However, the light output has quite a large spread due to the shape of the crystal and does not produce a focused light in one direction.

Structured scintillator crystals, such as CsI, have their crystals arranged more formally and tend to lie in parallel lines. This is due to the crystals being produced as long thin rods. As the end of the rod is the part of the crystal that faces the X-ray beam, it has a relatively small face plate area and therefore less chance of X-rays interacting with it. This results in a far more focused emission of light from the other side of the crystal facing the CCD array, but the overall amount of light produced tends to be much lower than with unstructured scintillators.

A secondary advantage of using structured crystals is that the shape of the crystal means incident X-rays have to fall directly onto the face plate. Any oblique rays (scattered radiation) are unlikely to cause the crystal to emit light eliminating the need for a secondary radiation grid enabling the radiation dose to be reduced (**Figure 6.14**).

Fortunately, the characteristics of both types of crystal are carefully matched to the recording systems.

Generally speaking, TFT systems work better with unstructured crystals and can utilize the high light output because they are closely coupled in a sandwich to the back of the scintillator crystal, so light is captured before it spreads out too much. Whereas CCD systems tend to use structured crystals as the more directional light, output is optically coupled through a mirror and lens (or optical fibres) and has to travel a relatively long distance to the CCD array.

Principles of Radiation Detection and Image Formation

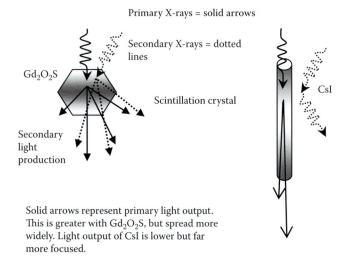

Primary X-rays = solid arrows

Secondary X-rays = dotted lines

Gd_2O_2S

Scintillation crystal

CsI

Secondary light production

Solid arrows represent primary light output. This is greater with Gd_2O_2S, but spread more widely. Light output of CsI is lower but far more focused.

Figure 6.14 Features of a scintillation crystal.

Indirect digital radiography using thin film transistor technology

The scintillator forms the top layer of a sandwich, the next layer being the photodiode layer. The light produced by the scintillator interacts with the photodiode which produces an electrical charge, which is proportional to the amount of light interacting with it.

The principles are similar to the single scintillation crystals/silicon photodiode multiplier detector described earlier in the chapter. The difference is that this is one large flat plate currently approaching 43 cm² (**Figure 6.15**).

How then do we get pixel densities of up to 400 mm² with IDR technology?

In contrast to CR technology, there is no latent image phase in the conventional sense (see below). The emitted electrical charge passes directly to the last part of the sandwich, the active matrix array (AMA) formed by the TFT charge collector layer covering the entire surface area of the photodiode. This layer is divided into an extremely fine grid of minute areas where the charge is collected and measured (**Figure 6.15**).

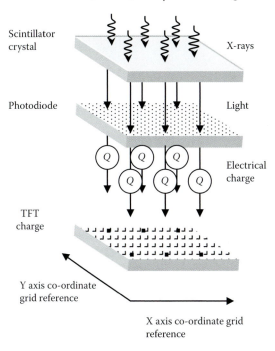

Figure 6.15 Diagram of an indirect radiography system.

The grid itself forms the raw data matrix with each area of the grid being given a co-ordinate reference in both the x and y axis.

Active matrix array in detail

The active matrix is essentially a very fine grid of transistors and capacitors held together in a thin layer (**Figure 6.16**).

It is the same size (in the x and y axis) as the scintillator crystal and photodiode layers that sit above it. The matrix itself will directly form the pixels in the resultant image. The grid will contain as many areas, known as detector elements (dels), as required for adequate resolution. Earlier we considered a resolution of ten line pairs per millimetre equating to a pixel density of 400 mm^2. This means that for full resolution images to be produced, the TFT charge collector will need to have

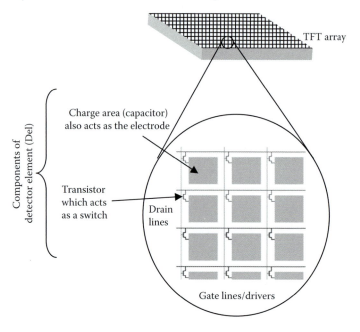

TFT array

Charge area (capacitor) also acts as the electrode

Components of detector element (Del)

Transistor which acts as a switch

Drain lines

Gate lines/drivers

Figure 6.16 Diagram of an active matrix array.

at least 400 dels (each containing a transistor and capacitor) for every mm^2 as well.

We also said earlier that no latent image is formed. This is true in the conventional sense as no relatively long-term latent image is formed. However, the electrical charge from the photodiode is connected to the electrode of the TFT and creates a short-term latent charge in the capacitor of the individual TFT dels to be stored, but it is only held for a fraction of a second. This is because a very short time later, the gate of the transistor for a particular del is switched on allowing the charge to be released and read from the TFT's drain line. In reality, this is not done 1 del at a time, many dels are turned on in a co-ordinated sequence with multiple readings being taken and digitised simultaneously, something known as 'multiplexing'.

In **Figure 6.16**, the columns and rows of the array form the gate and drain lines. Following an exposure, electronic circuits energise the gates of the transistors in the entire column. This causes a charge to be released from every del in the column with their charges flowing down individual drain lines (rows). This results in a specific amount of charge for every del in that column which is equivalent to the radiation that interacted with it. The next column is then energised and another set of charges flow down the drain lines and so on. This is done extremely quickly as it only requires the circuits to be switched electronically enabling us to obtain all the information from the entire matrix in just over a second.

Every del in the entire array will have an individual value attributed to it which is representative of the amount of radiation that interacted with it during exposure. This is digitised and displayed on a monitor in less than 10 seconds.

Information quoted about a particular TFT array often refers to what is known as the 'fill factor'. Essentially this is the proportion of sensitive area (charge collection area) against the dead areas of the array which includes the tiny electronic circuits (gate, drain, transistor and capacitor electronics) between the collection areas. A fill factor of 1 means the entire area is sensitive, but such a system cannot exist with current technology as we will always need the associated electronics to send the information, creating the dead area.

There is a manufacturing limit on how small we can make the electronics which are similar sized, regardless of the resolution of the array. This means that the sensitive area is relatively large in comparison to the electronics for a low resolution array, in the region of 0.8 but is more likely to be around 0.5, for high resolution systems. This means that only 50 per cent of the array is sensitive to radiation in the higher resolution system, the rest is filled with electronic circuits. This obviously reduces the DQE with the higher resolution system, it also effectively limits the spatial resolution that TFT systems can achieve.

Indirect digital radiography using charged coupled device technology

In many respects, CCD technology produces very similar results to TFT technology. The difference lies in the physical size of the CCD array which is not big enough to cover the planar dimension of the scintillator.

In some respects, even though CCDs are solid-state detectors, they actually work in a similar way to ionisation chambers except they are designed to work with photons of light rather than be directly exposed to X-radiation. However, X-rays will also affect them, which is why they are carefully positioned to avoid X-rays interacting with them.

Their main advantages include high spatial resolution, wide dynamic range, low electronic noise and linear response.

As they are sensitive to light, it also means they do not need the photodiode layer of the TFT system, as they can produce a signal directly from the light output of the scintillator.

The photon of light from the scintillator strikes the surface of the CCD del and is enough to eject an electron from its orbit. A potential difference is applied across the individual CCD del which causes the ions to move to different areas of the del where they are collected.

This is where the technology varies to other designs. Rather than the signal being read here it transfers its charge to its neighbouring del. While at the same time its neighbour also transfers its charge, and so on, across the whole array, hence the name 'charged coupled devices'. This happens in both the x and y axis at the same time producing a serial signal which is collected at one corner of the array. If this serial signal is then calculated against a time line, it is possible to determine exactly from where the signal originated within the array.

One reason for designing the array in this way is that we do not need signal wires similar to the gates and drains of TFT technology running throughout the array and therefore the space between the dels is much smaller, meaning they have far better resolution with a CCD pixel size of around 0.10–0.14 µm.

Typical high resolution CCD systems have 4000 × 4000 dels, giving a total of 16 000 000 dels (effectively a 16 mega pixel system), a similar number of dels to those in TFT arrays. However, in order to maintain high charge coupling ratios required for serial transmission, CCD arrays are limited to relatively small sizes, with typical overall dimensions of only 4 × 4 cm.

This means the light output covering an area of 43 cm^2 from the scintillator has to be reduced to cover the photosensitive areas of the CCD which is only 4 cm^2. Consequently, even though the CCD pixel is around 0.10–0.14 µm, this is the demagnified pixel size of CCD array;

the actual raw data pixel represents an area in the region of between 100 and 200 μm and this is the true resolution of the system.

One of the design considerations of these systems is how to connect and where to place the CCD array. In addition to light, CCDs are also sensitive to X-rays. Any X-rays interacting with the CCD could affect the charge coupling and create a false signal. Therefore, the array cannot be positioned in line with the scintillator crystal where X-rays may interact with it.

There are two ways to achieve this: one way is to use fibre optical tapers; the other way is to use a mirror and optical lens arrangement.

Charged coupled device coupling via optical fibre

Figure 6.17 shows six tapering optical fibres. In reality, if we wanted to manufacture such a system to cover the full 43 cm² area of the scintillator and match it to the CCD array, we would need 4000 × 4000, a total of 16 000 000 tapers. Due to the relative expense of having this many fibres, it would be prohibitively expensive for use in a general X-ray room.

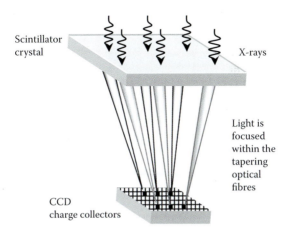

Figure 6.17 Diagram of a charged couple device (CCD) coupling via optical fibre.

However, there are some systems that use a modified scaled down version of this technology. Two of the most common systems will be briefly outlined. Both of the systems use what is known as 'slot scan techniques' to produce images.

Slot scan chest radiography

The first system is a dedicated chest X-ray system where the X-ray beam is tightly collimated to an area of around 1 cm high × 43 cm wide. The corresponding imaging system uses a 1 cm high scintillating crystal, again 43 cm wide. The scintillator is attached to a series of CCD arrays connected by optical fibres, but as the coverage is only 1 cm × 43 cm, the number of fibres required is much less than the number required to cover 43 cm^2 making such a system now financially viable (**Figure 6.18**).

How then do they cover the full 43 cm^2 required for a chest examination?

These systems essentially scan the chest to produce the image. The X-ray beam and detectors move from the top of the chest to the bottom during exposure with a 1 cm moving strip covering the width of the chest as it moves down the chest; this is all done in a single breath hold.

The advantages of this technique include a two- to four-fold reduction in dose over conventional CR and DR systems, very high resolution

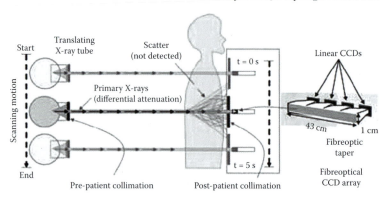

Linear CCD slot-scan array large image acquisition

Figure 6.18 Linear charged couple device (CCD) slot scan array large image acquisition.

and also benefits from low levels of noise and little scatter due to rod-shaped CsI scintillator crystals acting a little like a secondary radiation grid. It is currently regarded as one of the most effective systems for radiography of the chest.

The only real disadvantage is that the equipment is only really capable of this one job and would only warrant being installed in a dedicated chest facility.

The second system is a dedicated digital mammography system which uses a batch of fibreoptic tapers linked to a CCD detector array with 8192 × 400 channels. It operates in a very similar way to the chest slot scan systems, but everything is scaled down to produce a very fine scanning strip of 1 cm × 22 cm. Due to the small size of CCD it actually needs four CCD arrays to cover the 22 cm width. Each CCD has a matrix of 2048 wide × 400 high, by adding the four arrays together. This give us a matrix which is 8192 channels wide × 400 channels high. It takes about 6 seconds for the beam to scan the breast, but the images produced exhibit exceptional image quality together with a relatively low radiation dose.

However, for the reasons previously discussed, this technology for all its benefits does not suit large area single exposure techniques required for most body areas. This means the optical coupling method discussed below is the only viable option for general radiography.

Charged coupled devices optically coupled by a mirror and high quality lens

The light output from the scintillator is bent through 90° by a high quality mirror, it is then reduced in size and focused by a very high quality optical lens on to the 4 cm CCD array (**Figure 6.19**).

This is potentially a very effective system, but it does suffer from a few disadvantages. One issue relates to the size of optics and mirror which require a relatively large space within the X-ray equipment, meaning it is only possible to incorporate this type of technology into specifically designed X-ray couches and upright imaging systems.

Other issues are related to demagnification and optical maintenance. Demagnification is inherent in the system design and is basically the effect of taking a relatively large scintillator light output and minimising it to fit the size of the CCD and then enlarging it again to view on

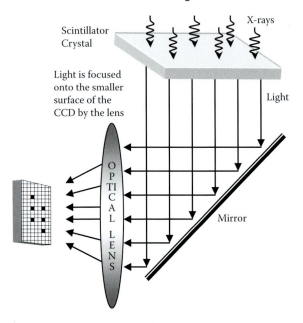

Figure 6.19 Charged Couple Device (CCD) system and optical mirror.

a workstation, which subsequently reduces image quality. The other issue of optical maintenance is related to anything that degrades the effectiveness of the optics, such as dust or alignment problems interfering with the fidelity of the transmission of light.

Direct digital radiography

One system that serves as an example is provided in **Figure 6.20**.

These detectors work in a similar way to ionisation chambers. When incident radiation passes into the sensitive volume, it causes electrons to be liberated from their orbits forming positive and negative ions to carry the charge from one electrode to the other. These are attached to their respective electrodes creating a current which the image acquisition system, in contrast to IDR, converts the X-rays to an electrical signal without the need for first converting it to light. With solid-state semi-conductor materials, the incident radiation produces electrons and holes in pairs that carry the charge.

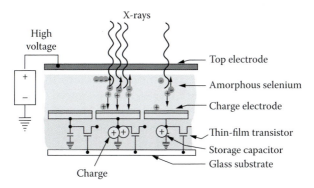

Figure 6.20 Direct digital radiography (DDR) system.

The top surface of the imaging system is made of a thin metal coating and forms one of the electrodes. X-rays pass through this first layer quite easily into the layer below the dielectric layer (electrical insulator), again relatively unhindered. They then pass into the next layer, which is a solid-state semi-conductor material where the interactions take place. The X-rays interact with the atoms in the semi-conductor layer and form electron hole pairs in proportion to the quantity and quality of incident X-rays falling on it. The last layer is a TFT array that also forms the other electrode. This TFT electrode is not a single area, but is actually composed of many minute electrodes formed by the sensitive areas of every del in the TFT which directly form the image matrix.

The electrodes of the face plate and those forming the TFT have an opposite charge applied to them in the order of a few kilovolts, so one will be positively charged and the other negatively charged. It does not necessarily matter which of the plates is positively charged and which is negatively charged, but different polarities do cause the systems to have slightly different properties which are exploited differently by different manufacturers. It is beyond the scope of this book to explore this in more detail.

Electron hole pair refers to the electric and the remaining positive atom which both have an equal and opposite charge

Following exposure, electron hole pairs are created in the semi-conductor layer by interactions of the X-ray beam. Due to the high kilovoltage, the electrons immediately flow towards the positive electrode while the positive atom flows towards the negative electrode. The high kilovoltage also inhibits the recombination of the electrons and holes. The electrodes are carefully aligned making use of the high kV to create field lines that will funnel the ions pairs directly towards their respective electrode plates with very little lateral spread of information. This ensures few if any ions fall outside the del on to the interspace (or dead space created by the associated electronics, the gates and drain lines), resulting in excellent spatial resolution. The electrodes on the underneath of the semi-conductor layer are connected directly to or from part of a matching TFT array which essentially has the same role as with IDR using TFT technology.

As with IDR technology, the size of the dels in these TFT systems is again the main limiting factor in resolution. However, in addition to this being limited by the dead space, the minute electrodes in this application of TFT technology also have to be a certain size in order to cope with a relatively high kV.

The main semi-conductor currently in use with these systems is amorphous selenium (a-Se). This substance can have issues where the charges become trapped at the electrode interface making it difficult to fully clear these charges before the next exposure resulting in remnants of the previous exposure affecting the latest image. Some systems perform detector 'relaxation' following an exposure to release trapped charges within the substrate. This phenomenon gets worse with time as the a-Se naturally tries to crystallise with ever increasing effects on its semi-conducting properties.

It is worth noting that newer manufacturing techniques, such as doping a-Se with arsenic, have reduced these effects significantly. Another substance, amorphous silicon (a-Si), is also being developed and is used in a similar way and exhibits very similar properties.

So which is the better system CR/DR or DI?

The main supporters of CR would argue it has the greatest versatility of any system and can be used with unmodified equipment as well as being available in different cassette sizes, while proponents of DR argue for the speed of the system.

In terms of resolution, it is possible to alter this with CR, but most current research suggests that DR has the advantage. Recent studies also suggest that if we require resolutions less than 200 µm, then a-Se performs better, but for resolutions of more than 200 µm, then a-Si panels may perform better.

In terms of dose we suggest the reader looks at texts explaining these matters in more detail.

DIGITAL FLUOROSCOPIC SYSTEMS

Image intensifier linked to charged coupled device

Early digital fluoroscopy systems tended to revolve around an analogue image intensifier (II) linked to a CCD camera. The CCD output was converted to a digital output via an analogue to digital converter.

Images need to be produced at a rate of 30 or more frames per second in order to produce a smooth real-time moving image. As CCDs use fast serial data collection together with extremely fast transmission speeds, these frame rates are easily achieved. CCDs also benefit from extremely low inherent noise and can produce good image quality even from the relatively low exposure used during the fluoroscopy mode, as well as extra low-dose pulse techniques.

For these reasons, CCD using an image intensifier became the dominant system and this type of technology is still the most widespread in clinical use. Even so, there are some issues: it requires a large housing and its image is distorted to some degree by the signal amplification that takes place inside the image intensifier. As a result of these inherent limitations, this technology is now being replaced by the flat panel technologies.

Fluoroscopic flat panel detectors

Initially, there were issues associated with using flat panel technology to produce real-time images. The systems suffered from lag and slow refresh rates, which although not an issue for still radiographic images, is a real issue in fluoroscopy mode. The system must collect all the signals from all detector elements, for each frame, within a thirtieth of a second; this is extremely difficult to achieve and places high demands on the switching characteristics of the components that make up the TFTs, as well as the speed of the charge amplifiers and digitisers of the output stage. The result is that early systems were not able to achieve the 30+ frames per second required for smooth motion real-time imaging.

The second issue relates to radiation dose during fluoroscopic examinations. While flat panel detectors are comparable in terms of dose with other systems for still images they initially gave relatively high doses when used for moving fluoroscopic images. Traditional fluoroscopic systems including digital image intensifier systems using CCD technology could produce images of good quality using relatively low mA. Image quality was still acceptable with even more aggressive dose reduction techniques where the beam was pulsed during fluoroscopic mode. This allowed a significant lowering of the overall dose the patient received for an examination.

Unfortunately, early flat panel technology did not respond very well to the low quantity of incident radiation during standard fluoroscopy mode and consequently suffered very poor signal-to-noise ratios. The signal-to-noise situation was even worse with pulsed low-dose techniques.

Recent developments in flat panel technology using modified formulations of scintillator and photodiode materials, as well as introducing overcharging protection circuits, help in significantly reducing lag, speeding up refresh rates, as well as responding better to low-dose fluoroscopic techniques, enabling much better overall image quality. They do not suffer from geometric distortion, such as pincushion and S-shaped distortion, offering excellent image uniformity. Current systems also benefit from an image area of up to 43 cm^2 and art therefore able to cover the commonly used techniques and examinations of the entire body, something early systems also struggled with. This has led to more widespread uptake of flat panel technology for fluoroscopic purposes.

Solid-state X-ray image intensifier

There has been much research into the technology of the solid-state X-ray image intensifier (SSXII) which is based on a technology called electron multiplying CCD (EMCCD).

SSXII is essentially a series of modified CCD arrays which are butted together forming a much larger array (43 cm²). The modifications include an on-chip amplifier which removes the need for a traditional image intensifier. A CsI scintillator is still used with a traditional analogue image intensifier, but instead of the light being amplified by the intensifier it is used directly by the EMCCD.

The system is very similar in design to the fibreoptic coupled CCD systems used in slot scan techniques discussed earlier in this chapter. The light output of the CsI scintillator in response to an exposure is coupled to the EMCCD. By using optical fibres, this system has a much higher resolution than the three line pairs per millimetre (lp/mm) available with both the CCDII and flat panel detectors (FPD) and is able to provide an effective pixel size of 32 μm. It has all the advantages of the flat panel systems and also benefits from no lag or ghosting. Signal to noise ratios are exceptional; all CCDs benefit from extremely low noise levels, but in addition EMCCDs also benefit from a built-in amplifier, enabling them to detect tiny signals.

Reference

Lança L, Silva A. Digital radiography detectors – a technical overview: part 2. *Radiography* 2009; **15**: 134–8.

MCQs

1. **The DQE is:**
   a. Essentially based on its overall signal-to-noise ratio (SNR) when compared against a theoretical ideal detector.
   b. Not affected by spatial frequency.
   c. Not a variable as signal values change in response to changes in exposure.
   d. Essentially based on the modular transfer function (MTF) when compared against a theoretical ideal detector.

2. **Indirect systems:**
   a. May be CR or IDR
   b. Are just CR
   c. Are just IDR
   d. May be CR, IDR or DDR.

3. **The following are characteristics of structured scintillation crystals:**
   a. They have high output in comparison to unstructured scintillation crystals and light is in a more forward direction.
   b. They have low output in comparison to unstructured scintillation crystals and light is in a more forward direction.
   c. They have low output in comparison to unstructured scintillation crystals and light is in a less forward direction.
   d. They have high output in comparison to unstructured scintillation crystals and light is in a less forward direction.

4. **TFT systems work better with:**
   a. Unstructured crystals due to their higher light output
   b. Structured crystals as the light output is more directional
   c. Unstructured crystals as the light output is more directional
   d. Unstructured crystals due to their lower light output.

5. **TFT arrays are:**
   a. Usually connected to the scintillator crystals by optical fibres
   b. Optically connected to the scintillator by a lens and mirror system.
   c. Directly connected to the back of the scintillator
   d. Attached to the output phosphor of a digital fluoroscopy image intensifier.

6. **Which of the following materials is used in systems that directly convert X-rays to electrical signal without the intermediate conversion to light?**
   a. Gadolinium oxisulphide (Gd_2O_2S)
   b. Caesium iodide (CsI)
   c. Amorphous selenium (a-Se)
   d. Barium fluoro-halide:europium activated/doped (Ba F Br_x I $_{1-x}$:Eu).

7. **The electrodes in a DDR system are formed by the face plate and those forming the TFT. Why do they have an opposite charge applied to them in the order of a few kilovolts, so one will be positively charged and the other negatively charged?**
   a. To create field lines in which the light can travel between electrodes
   b. To create field lines which inhibit the recombination of the electrons and holes

    c. To create field lines to increase signal, but they also create a small amount of interference which causes the signal to spread

    d. To create field lines in which the light can travel to the electrodes.

8. **Define the fill factor as related to the TFT array.**

    a. This is the ratio of the thickness of the sensitive layer in comparison to the whole thickness of the array.

    b. This is the proportion of electronic circuits to the thickness of the sensitive volume.

    c. Ratio of the number of live detector elements against the number of dead detector element in an array.

    d. Is the proportion of sensitive area (charge collection area) against the dead areas of the array which includes the tiny electronic circuits.

9. **What is the minimum number of frames in order to produce a smooth real-time moving image?**

    a. 30 frames per second

    b. 10 frames per second

    c. 20 frames per second

    d. 50 frames per second.

10. **Early designs of flat panel technology used to produce real-time images were associated with:**

    a. Exceptional temporal resolution, but relatively low signal output

    b. Exceptional temporal resolution, but required relatively high exposures

    c. Lag and slow refresh rates

    d. Poor temporal resolution, but benefited from relatively low exposure requirements.

CHAPTER 7
IMAGE QUALITY

INTRODUCTION

It is essential that any practitioner understands the principles involved in producing and assessing diagnostic images. Images must be produced with the lowest radiation dose consistent with diagnostic quality (ALARP (as low as reasonably practicable) principle). The practitioner therefore needs to understand how to adjust the factors affecting image quality to ensure the images answer the diagnostic question. Image quality is subjective (it depends on the skills of the observer) and may be difficult to define, however, an optimum quality image enables the observer to make an accurate diagnosis. Poor quality images are easier to define as they have a poor signal-to-noise ratio, poor spatial resolution and detract from the process of extracting information.

There are characteristics of an image which may be evaluated and this enables the practitioner to determine the diagnostic quality of an image.

These characteristics include:

- The positioning of the patient, X-ray beam and detector
- Collimating and centring of the beam to the area of interest
- Precise patient positioning with the area under examination parallel to the detector
- Ensuring the patient is comfortable and still to minimise movement.
- The data acquired by the detector
- Quantity and quality of photons which pass through the patient without attenuation (brightness and contrast)
- Scattered photons (noise)
- The display system used to view the image
- Monitor size and matrix size

- Software processing applied to the raw data.
- Viewing conditions (background illumination).

Learning objectives

The student should be able to:
- Understand and explain the principles of producing and assessing images for their image quality.
- Explain the factors which contribute to radiation dose and image quality.

GEOMETRY OF IMAGING

All radiographic images are larger than the object being X-rayed. This magnification is due to the geometry of imaging. The ideal situation is to have:

- The object being imaged parallel to the X-ray beam and the image receptor.
- The radiation beam at right angles to the object.
- A long focus to receptor distance and small object to receptor distance

This minimises the distortion of the image and the magnification of the unsharpness in the image.

The ideal conditions to produce radiographic images are shown in **Figure 7.1**.

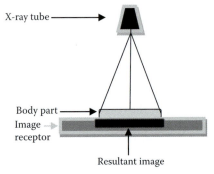

Figure 7.1 Ideal positioning for X-ray imaging.

The object should be as close to the image receptor as possible. As the object moves away from the image receptor the magnification increases. This makes the object bigger but also magnifies any unsharpness in the image.

The positioning of the patient (geometry) to produce the image has a direct relationship on the quality of that image.

Figure 1.2 in Chapter 1, Overview of image production, is a diagrammatic representation of image production and shows that a penumbra (unsharpness) is formed with any image that is produced from a finite source (focal spot). The diagram uses a large distance between the object and image receptor to illustrate the principle of penumbra. In practice, the amount of geometric unsharpness (Ug) in an image is small and may be much less than 0.4 mm (the point at which we begin to perceive unsharpness on an otherwise optimum image).

Measurement of the penumbra (Ug) is a straightforward calculation using similar triangles. Figure 1.1 in Chapter 1, for example, demonstrates the diagrammatic representation of similar triangles. It is possible to calculate the unsharpness in an image of a finger due to geometric unsharpness. The formula is:

$$Ug = \frac{Focal\ spot\ size \times ORD}{FRD}$$

To calculate the penumbra you need to know all the factors on the right side of the equation. For example, if the:

- Focal spot size is 0.3 mm.
- The focus receptor distance (FRD) is 110 cm.
- The object receptor distance (ORD) is 1 cm.

The unsharpness is calculated as only 0.001 mm, which is negligible and looks sharp to the observer. The values used here are typical in radiography.

When undertaking an X-ray of the lumbar spine, the geometric unsharpness is much larger. For example, if the:

- Focal spot size is 1 mm.
- FRD is 110 cm.
- ORD is 30 cm.

The unsharpness is calculated at 0.27 mm, which is approaching an image which the observer would perceive as blurred. Other factors, such as movement, and the resolution of the monitor will also increase this level of unsharpness.

Magnification and distortion

If the object being imaged is not parallel to the image receptor, it will be magnified, however, different aspects will be magnified differently and this will produce distortion. This may be elongation or foreshortening of the image. **Figure 7.2** shows the set up for producing a distorted image and **Figure 7.3** shows a deliberately elongated image of the scaphoid which aids in the diagnosis of a fracture.

The distance between the patient and the image receptor (ORD) should be as short as possible. For practical reasons, the FRD is usually 110 cm for techniques on the X-ray table and 180 cm for erect chest and cervical spine work. If possible, the object is in contact with the image receptor, however, using a Bucky assembly increases magnification of the image, but may be necessary to reduce scatter and improve the contrast of the image. Practically, the mechanism which moves the grid and houses the Potter–Bucky is kept as small as possible.

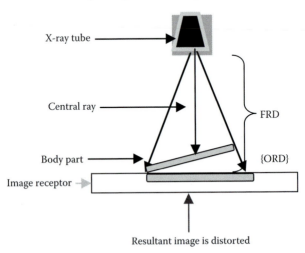

Figure 7.2 Set-up with variable ORD, which will give a distorted image.

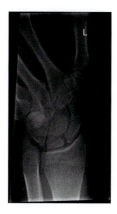

Figure 7.3 Elongated scaphoid projection.

Signal-to-noise ratio

Image quality may be assessed by the signal-to-noise ratio. The signal is the useful information from the patient being imaged and noise is anything which detracts from accessing the information. Useful information is derived from photoelectric interactions within the patient (absorption by dense body structures and no minimal absorption in air or instead of low density structures). Noise is derived from Compton scatter. The image receptor does not have the ability to determine the origin of scattered photons and there is also electrical noise from the system. Radiographic images that have a signal level which is high compared to the noise will enable structures to be clearly seen, but if the signal level is similar to or less than the noise level the structure will become obliterated.

Images produced by X-rays are often a compromise between obtaining a perfect signal and reducing the noise. The production of images is constrained by a number of factors including the radiation dose level and each component of the imaging chain, e.g. when imaging radiosensitive areas gonads, areas with red bone marrow, there is a constraint of minimising the radiation dose to that area. Extremities of the human body are less radiosensitive and images with higher dose and better definition may be reasonably acquired.

Use of a grid will also enhance contrast by removing scattered photons before they reaches the detector. The increased contrast by the use of a grid must be justified by the value of the practitioner, as using a grid will increase the dose proportionally by the grid factor.

Unsharpness

Unsharpness of an image is related to:

- The geometry of the imaging system
- Focal spot size
- Relationship (distance) between, focus, patient and detector.
- Intrinsic sharpness of the detector employed
- Subject contrast
- The quality and resolution of imaging system (film screen combination or video display unit (VDU))
- Beam quality (kV)
- Scatter (obscures the ability to observe sharpness)
- Movement unsharpness (usually patient movement).

In order to determine the image quality the image must be reasonably sharp. Blurring will reduce the image quality and also reduce the diagnostic quality of the image. The sharpness of a system is best characterised in terms of its modulation transfer function (MTF).

Movement unsharpness

Movement unsharpness should be kept to a minimum by careful radiographic technique. Making the patient comfortable, giving them precise instructions on breath-holding and practising the procedure may all help reduce movement unsharpness. Using short exposure times also helps reduce blur in the image. Exposure times as low as 0.001 s for a chest radiograph enables the practitioner to ensure minimum movement even in paediatrics.

Resolution of the imaging system

This will be covered in more detail in other chapters of this book. However, it should be noted that the smallest exposure compatible with diagnostic quality should be used. When determining the quality required in an image, the practitioner must be aware of what structures they need to define. An image to determine the position of bones in a plaster cast following an orthopaedic reduction needs less resolution than the original image to diagnose the fracture. Ideally, the smaller of the foci of the X-ray tube should be used (fine focus), but if this does not enable a short exposure time to be used on a patient likely to move, the practitioner may need to use a broad focus. This is another example of where the practitioner needs to make a decision which is a compromise between the ideal conditions and getting a diagnostic image.

Spatial resolution

Spatial resolution refers to the ability of the imaging system to represent distinct anatomic features within the object being imaged. It may be defined as the ability of the system to distinguish neighbouring features of an image from each other and is related to sharpness. The maximum spatial resolution of an image is defined by pixel size and spacing. Pixel size affects the system resolution and varies between systems. Detective quantum efficiency (DQE) combines spatial resolution (MTF) and image noise to provide a measure of the signal-to-noise ratio. The sharpness of an imaging detector or system is best characterised in terms of its MTF.

Measurement of unsharpness in an image

The sharpness of the image can be measured using a test tool (resolution) or by viewing the image and determining if fine structures can be visualized (definition). The resolution can be determined by measuring the ability of the imaging system to resolve the smallest object in the test tool and is expressed in line pairs per millimetre (lp/mm). This is perhaps an abstract concept to illustrate sharpness and it would be more sensible to determine the definition within the image, e.g. can I see the bony trabecular?

Again however, definition within the image is subjective and depends on a number of factors including the resolution of the monitor, viewing conditions and the experience of the practitioner viewing the image.

Viewing digital images

All digital images have a look-up table (LUT) applied to the raw data. The computer software enhances the image and displays the data with an 'optimum' brightness and contrast.

Brightness and contrast

The brightness may be defined as the intensity of light that represents the individual pixels in the image. Brightness is controlled by the processing software and can be adjusted following image processing.

Digital systems generally have a linear response to exposure and a wide dynamic range. All digital images are 'auto-windowed' so the computer will automatically apply an algorithm to the data detected and provide the 'best' range of densities (contrast) and brightness.

Over- and underexposure is therefore not visually apparent and other means are necessary to determine if the optimum exposure has been used. These checks include:

- Evaluation of the exposure indicator (EI). The number allocated to the image should be in the range expected by the system, e.g.
  - Computed radiography (CR) system acceptable range is given as 1700–2300. The ideal exposure is 2000 (may vary slightly for different body parts).
  - Digital radiography (DR) system range is given as 200–800. The ideal exposure is 400.
- Evaluation of noise within the image due to underexposure (**Figure 7.4a**).
- Evaluation of 'burn through' due to gross overexposure (**Figure 7.4c**).

If the EI is consistently higher than recommended, the patient is being overexposed and receiving to high a radiation dose.

Figure 7.4 shows a range of images from a CR system. The images range from an optimum quality image (**Figure 7.4b**), an underexposed image (**Figure 7.4a**) and a grossly overexposed image (**Figure 7.4c**) as measured using the EI.

Optimum images can be obtained from a wide range of exposures and **Figures 7.4a** and **7.4c** show the extremes where the computer failed to adjust the image into the diagnostic range due to the extremes of over-/underexposure.

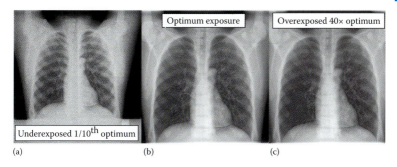

Figure 7.4 Underexposed image (a); optimum image (b); and overexposed image (c).

Contrast may be defined as a measure of the relative brightness difference between two locations (area or pixels) in an image. The contrast of an imaging system is described by the characteristic response curve of the system.

The X-ray beam is attenuated in the patient depending on the energy of the X-ray beam (quality) and the total exposure (mA and kVp). These factors were critical using film screen technology, however, when the image is 'auto-windowed'. In digital systems, these factors are less important and images taken at 60 and 110 kV may have similar brightness and contrast levels when displayed and viewed on a monitor (especially with the mA adjusted to compensate for the change in kV). **Figure 7.5** demonstrates images with similar contrast and brightness auto-windowed by CR system.

Note: If a range of exposures exists for producing a diagnostic image, the practitioner should always select the total exposure with the lowest radiation dose.

When imaging variations within the human body, there is a natural subject contrast. This varies depending on thickness of the patient and the area of the body, i.e.

- The thorax has high inherent contrast because adjacent areas have large differences in density of structures (dense heart muscle surrounded by air).
- The abdomen has low inherent contrast with adjacent areas having a similar atomic number (muscle, fat and organs).

The subject contrast cannot be altered, however, the auto-windowing can modify the image to improve the brightness and contrast before the image is displayed and the practitioner can also 'window' the image during post-processing. Both these processes may be able to 'create' a diagnostic image from poor raw data.

Generally, if the image appears 'optimum' for both 50 & 100 kV, the high kV should be used as it delivers a lower radiation dose.

Effect of scatter on contrast

Scattered radiation reaching the detects reduces the contrast of any image as it does not carry useful information, but does create a signal on the detector. The effect can be minimised by:

- Reducing the production of scatter
  - Close collimation to the area of interest
  - Displacement of the body part (used in mammography)
- Preventing the scatter reaching the detector
  - Using a grid or Bucky assembly
  - Using an air gap.

Scattered radiation should therefore be minimised by the practitioner.

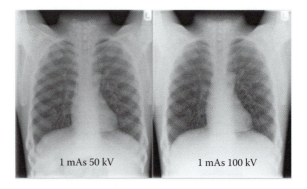

Figure 7.5 Optimum images taken at 50 and 100 kV.

MCQs

1. You are producing an image of the spine. The focus receptor distance (FRD) is 100 cm and the spine is 20 cm from the imaging plane. The spine is 40 cm long. What is the length of the spine in the image?
   a. 50 cm
   b. 5 cm
   c. 44 cm
   d. 40 cm.

2. Which of the following factors do not directly affect the sharpness of an image?
   a. Focus receptor distance (FRD)
   b. Focal spot size
   c. Scattered radiation
   d. Object receptor distance (ORD).

3. Which of the following factors produces an optimum image?
   a. Longest FRD practicable
   b. Smallest focus available
   c. Close contact between the patient and detector
   d. All of the above.

4. Calculate the penumbra if focus is 0.2 × 0.2 mm, the FRD is 110 and ORD is 2 cm.
   a. 3.6 mm
   b. 0.36 mm
   c. 0.036 mm
   d. 0.0036 mm.

5. Optimum images have:
   a. High signal-to-noise ratio
   b. Low signal-to-noise ratio
   c. Equal signal-to-noise ratio
   d. High electrical noise.

6. Which of the following arrangements produces an image with minimal unsharpness?
   a. Short FRD and long ORD
   b. Short FRD and short ORD
   c. Long FRD and short ORD
   d. Object parallel to the detector.

7. Which of the following factors cause noise in an image?
   a. Photoelectric absorption
   b. Transmitted photons
   c. Compton scatter
   d. Using a grid.

8. Spatial resolution is the ability of the system to:
   a. Minimize radiation dose
   b. Represent distinct anatomical detail
   c. Reduce blurring
   d. Reduce noise.

9. Which anatomical area has the highest inherent contrast?
   a. Thorax
   b. Abdomen
   c. Hand
   d. Pelvis.

10. If a range of exposures produces a diagnostic image you should:
    a. Use the lowest kV
    b. Use the highest kV
    c. Use the exposure which gives the lowest radiation dose
    d. Use the lowest mA.

CHAPTER 8
RADIATION DOSE AND EXPOSURE INDICATORS

INTRODUCTION

The radiation exposure from diagnostic X-rays is the largest man-made source of radiation exposure to the general population worldwide. Man-made exposure contributes about 14 per cent of the total annual exposure from all sources. Although diagnostic X-rays provide great benefits, their use involves some small risk of developing cancer. The aim of this chapter is to give the practitioner an understanding of the basic ways radiation dose can be measured and expressed to the patient and other staff. It will also explain exposure indicators used with digital systems. It is essential that any practitioner operating within an imaging department and using ionising radiation has a sound base for their knowledge. You need to comprehend and be able to explain the factors affecting radiation dose, methods of measuring dose and how dose may be expressed using exposure indicators.

> **Learning objectives**
> The student should be able to:
> - State and explain the factors affecting radiation dose and the methods of measuring dose.
> - Understand and explain the principles of exposure indicators.

RADIATION DOSE

Radiation may be measured and expressed in several ways. These account for the different sensitivities of the body tissues. For the purposes of this book, we will only consider X-rays and γ-radiation which have identical properties.

Detection and measurement of radiation

There are several methods used to detect and measure radiation. Some are more sensitive and accurate than others, but they all work on the principle of ionisation of a material and then measuring the effect. The methods include:

- Direct ionisation
  - An ionisation chamber
  - Free air ionisation chamber
  - Thimble dosimeter
  - Dose area product (DAP) metres
  - Automatic exposure devices (AED) used to terminate exposures rather than measure the dose.
  - Geiger–Muller tube
  - Gold leaf electroscope (Quartz fibre dosimeter).
- Luminescence
  - Photostimulated luminescence (PSL) resulting in the emission of blue light in an amount proportional to the original X-ray irradiation
  - Phosphors in screens used with film
- Scintillation
  - Scintillation probe and gamma camera
- Exposure of photographic film
  - X-ray film
  - Radiation film badges
- Thermoluminescenct dosimeters (TLD)
  - Dosimeters for whole body doses and separate monitors for small body parts

- Semi-conductor detection
  - Gamma camera
  - Flat panel detectors
  - Fluoroscopy units

Ionisation of air

Air in its normal state is considered to be a good electrical insulator as it does not contain any conduction electrons. However, if air is exposed to X- or γ-radiation, some of the photons of radiation will release electrons from the atoms in the air. This causes ionisation enabling the air to conduct electricity. The more radiation the air is exposed to, the more electrons emitted and the better able it is to conduct electric current. By measuring the electrons in the sample of air, the quantity of radiation causing the ionisation may be calculated/estimated.

The ionisation in air by the beam of radiation is proportional to the energy absorbed. The energy required to produce one ionisation in air is approximately 33 electron volts (eV). Therefore, if we have a homogenous beam X-rays at 60 kVp, this will produce about 1800 electrons. (This is a tiny amount compared to an electrical current of 1 picoamp, which is about 1 million electrons flowing through the conductor per second.)

Atomic numbers of air (7.6) and soft tissue (muscle) (7.4) are similar and therefore absorb about the same amount of energy. This means the mass absorption coefficients of air and soft tissue are very similar and by measuring the value in air, the value in tissue can be accurately estimated.

EXPOSURE

The traditional method of measuring the amount of ionisation in air was exposure. This measured the ratio of the total charge produced (of one sign, usually electrons) in a small volume of air. The unit of exposure for air is Coulombs per kilogram of air (C/kg). The unit of exposure only applies to X- and γ-radiation. The intensity (exposure rate) of a beam of X-rays can also be measured as the energy passing through unit area in unit time.

Absorbed dose

The Gray (Gy) is the SI unit of absorbed dose and is equivalent to the absorption of one joule of energy in a kilogram of a substance by ionising radiation. For X-rays and gamma radiation, the Gray equates to the Sievert (equivalent dose) as the quality factor (QF) for X- and γ-radiation is one.

The Gray is a large unit and, for normal radiation protection purposes, it is more common to use subunits like the:

- Microgray (μGy) is one millionth of a Gray (1×10^{-6})
- Milligray (mGy) is one thousandth of a Gray (1×10^{-3}).

Kerma dose is different from absorbed dose especially at high energies (up to 1 MeV) and roughly equal at low energies. The unit for kerma is joule per kilogram (Gy), which is the same as for absorbed dose. When a photon beam interacts with a medium, the photon interactions release electrons with kinetic energy into the medium (kerma) which then move on to deposit energy along ionisation tracks. The energy deposited by these electrons per unit mass is the absorbed dose. So 'kerma' is energy released and 'absorbed dose' is energy absorbed. The total absorbed energy delivered by the secondary electrons produced by a photon beam is the 'integral dose'. The integral dose attempts to describe energy deposition within the whole body.

Equivalent dose

Equivalent dose allows the effect of radiation exposure on human tissue to be determined. It relates the absorbed dose in human tissue to the effective biological damage of the radiation. Not all radiation has the same biological effect, even for the same amount of absorbed dose. The SI unit of equivalent dose is the Sievert (Sv) and represents the stochastic biological effect. The Sievert is a large unit and for normal radiation protection levels a series of prefixes are used:

- MicroSievert (μSv) is one millionth of a Sievert (1×10^{-6})
- MilliSievert (mSv) is one thousandth of a Sievert (1×10^{-3}).

To determine equivalent dose (Sv), you multiply absorbed dose (Gy) by a radiation weighting factor (W_R) that is unique to the type of radiation. The W_R takes into account that some kinds of radiation are inherently more dangerous to biological tissue, even if their 'energy deposition' levels are the same. For X-rays and gamma radiation, and electrons absorbed by human tissue, the W_R is 1.

To determine the dose in Sieverts from the dose in Grays, simply multiply by the W_R. This is obviously a simplification. The W_R approximates what otherwise would be a very complicated calculation. The values for W_R change periodically as new research refines the SBKs associated with radiation exposure.

Exposure occurs over time, of course. The more Sieverts absorbed in a unit of time, the more intense the exposure. So we express exposure as an amount over a specific time period, e.g. 5 milliSieverts per year. This is called the 'dosage rate'. In the UK, the dose rate from background radiation, the sum of all natural radiation, is about 2.5 millisieverts per year.

Effective dose

The probability of a harmful effect from radiation exposure depends on the part or parts of the body exposed. Some organs are more sensitive to radiation than others. A tissue weighting factor is used to take this into account. When an equivalent dose to an organ is multiplied by the tissue weighting factor for that organ, the result is the effective dose to that organ.

If more than one organ is exposed, then the effective dose, E, is the sum of the effective doses to all exposed organs (**Figure 8.1**).

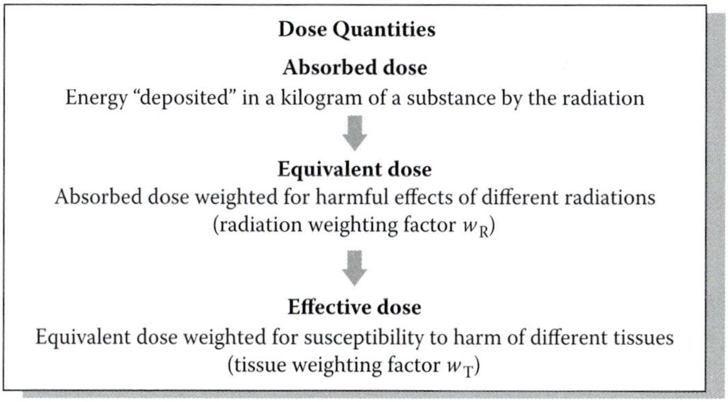

Dose Quantities

Absorbed dose
Energy "deposited" in a kilogram of a substance by the radiation

⬇

Equivalent dose
Absorbed dose weighted for harmful effects of different radiations
(radiation weighting factor w_R)

⬇

Effective dose
Equivalent dose weighted for susceptibility to harm of different tissues
(tissue weighting factor w_T)

Figure 8.1 Dose quantities and their relationship.

Linear energy transfer and relative biological effectiveness

When ionising radiation passes through tissue (a medium) it may inter-act with it and deposit energy along its path of travel. The average energy deposited per unit length is called the linear energy transfer (LET). The energy absorbed in tissue depends on the type of charged ionising par-ticle which is travelling through the medium and the type of medium. LET is measured in kiloelectron volts (KeV) per micron (10-6 m) and is an important factor in assessing potential tissue damage. For diagnos-tic beams the LET is considered relatively low. When diagnostic beams interact with tissue it causes damage by the production of free radicals which may cause damage to the DNA. High LET radiation eg alpha par-ticles are more destructive to biological tissue as they lose their energy in a shorter length of tissue and are more ionising.

Another consideration in dosimetry is the relative biological effec-tiveness (RBE) of radiation. This describes the relative ability of ionis-ing radiation to produce a biological reaction. RBE is not suitable for determining the biological effects in humans for all types of radiation but is similar for X-rays in the diagnostic range.

Quality factor for radiation

The same absorbed doses of different types of radiation cause a dif-ferent biological damage in tissue. X-rays, gamma radiation and beta particles all produce virtually the same biological effect on tissue for equal absorbed doses and are given a quality factor of 1. A *quality fac-tor* is used to adjust the dose equivalent of other types of radiation eg alpha particles have a quality factor of 20 and have a much greater effect on tissue.

Radiation monitors and personal monitoring

The principles of ionisation chambers are described in Chapter 6, Ionisation monitors may be used for dosimetry. Other types of per-sonal dosimeters used to monitor staff doses are:

- Radiation film badges, which use a double-sided film emulsion, and
- Thermoluminescen dosimeters, which are used for whole body doses or small body parts.

Thermoluminescent dosimeters (TLD)

The TLD card comprises two elements of lithium fluoride (LiF) mounted in an aluminium frame and has a uniquely numbered barcode that can be read automatically and the radiation dose can be measured. After readout, the card can be annealed to get rid of any residual reading and then reissued. A TLD card can go through this readout/anneal cycle more than 500 times.

TLD monitors are the most commonly used monitor. The badge is comprised of a TLD card (**Figure 8.2**), which is placed in a holder that incorporates a filter system. This allows the radiation type and energy to be determined. It is used to determine the whole body exposure of people who may be exposed to beta-, gamma- or X-rays. It can be worn for 4 to 12 week period wearing period depending on the work carried out and the risk to the operator. The extremity (or finger) TLD is used by anyone who may be exposed to significant doses to the fingers. The monitor consists of a small plastic sachet containing a TLD which can be chemically disinfected if necessary.

The doses are determined by the measurement of the light output from the TLD card. Thermoluminescent materials store energy inside their structure when they are irradiated, as electrons and holes are trapped in trapping centres due to crystaline defects. When that material is heated, electrons and the positive atom recombine, at luminescence centres, and thus light is emitted. The light is measured using a PMT (photomultiplier tube) inside the reader device. The photons which are emitted are in the visible region and they comprise the thermoluminescent (TL) signal.

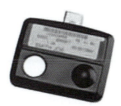

Figure 8.2 Thermoluminescence dosimeter badge.

Exposure indicators

Sometimes known as detector dose indicators (DDI), exposure indicators (EI) are used to provide feedback, in the form of a standard index, to operators of digital radiographic systems. This reflect the adequacy of the exposure that has reached the detector after every exposure event. Due to the very wide dynamic range of digital imaging systems, there is now little visual indication of exposure variation in the images displayed on the monitor. A digital image processing technique called 'histogram auto-ranging' is used in all systems to stop 'over- or under-exposure' from changing the lightness or darkness of the image. The International Commission for Radiation Protection (ICRP) decreed that all computed radiography (CR) and digital radiography (DR) systems must incorporate some form of exposure indicator. Their main fear was that dramatic overexposure might occur without the radiographer being aware of it, if they simply relied on the image as they were used to doing with film/screen systems.

The direct connection between the level of detector exposure and optical density is well established in film-screen radiology. This is not the case in digital radiography, where almost always, a constant image characteristic is achieved using automatic image processing. Consequently, deviations from the intended exposure, i.e. over- and underexposure, are not noticeable by a corresponding deviation in image brightness. While considerable underexposure results in an increased level of noise, the more alarming aspect (from a radiation protection point of view) is that overexposure cannot be recognised easily in the displayed image. The final brightness of the image is controlled not by the exposure to the detector, but by automatic image processing applied to the acquired raw data. Consequently, overexposed images may not necessarily be dark, and underexposed images may not appear light. This may be a new and confusing concept for operators of digital radiographic systems who are accustomed to screen-film imaging.

For more than a decade, the phenomenon of 'exposure creep' in photostimulable storage phosphor imaging has been reported. This is attributed to the fact that digital imaging systems can produce adequate image contrast over a much broader range of exposure levels than screen-film imaging systems. Average exposure levels tend to creep up over time if a clear indicator of exposure is not provided and routinely monitored. Techniques required to achieve optimal radiographic imaging in DR may be different from those used for film/screen imaging.

This broad dynamic range is one of the benefits of digital detectors. However, if the detector is underexposed higher noise levels may obscure the presence of subtle details in the image. Excessive detector exposures may produce high quality images with improved noise characteristics, but at the expense of increased patient dose.

The dynamic range for the chest X-ray is from 1 mAs and 70 kVp to 20 mAs and 110 kVp with all images of diagnostic quality (**Figure 8.3**).

The American Association of Physicists therefore recommended an exposure index for every image taken and a deviation index which indicates the amount the exposure varies from a designated aim point.

This will identify:

- Under- and over exposure
- Exposure distribution and exposure drift
- A basis for evaluation of new technology.

An index of detector exposure is appropriate because it reflects the noise content, and thus the signal-to-noise ratio in the image. For DR systems, the appropriate incident exposure is variable based on the desired signal-to-noise ratio rather than on the resulting optical density of a radiograph. Different digital detectors may require more or less radiation exposure to achieve the same noise content depending upon the detective quantum efficiency (DQE) of the detector technology in use.

The concept of an exposure indicator was adopted, however, there are currently over a dozen systems in place. Some manufacturers

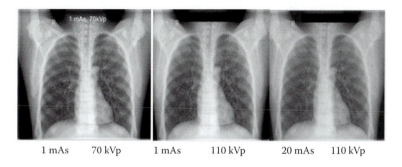

| 1 mAs | 70 kVp | 1 mAs | 110 kVp | 20 mAs | 110 kVp |

Figure 8.3 Dynamic range of digital radiography for a chest image.

System	Exposure Indicator	Target parameters for extremities at 60kV	Target parameter for the rest of the body at 80kV	Change by factor of 2
Kodak	Exposure Index	1850	2060	300
Fuji	Sensitivity number (S)	300	150	30
Agfa	Log median value (LgM)	1.85	2.06	0.3

Figure 8.4 Exposure indicators for four systems.

have different systems for their CR and DR systems. Unfortunately, the indicator for exposure drift was not adopted.

The exposure indicators for the three manufacturers available in the UK are shown in **Figure 8.4**. As can be seen, they used three different names for the indicators and almost different methods for indicating the correct index. This is certainly not what the regulators had in mind.

As can be seen in the table the manufacturers recommend target values for 60 kV & 80 kV exposures. Extremities exposed at 60 kVp have a different target than exposures for the rest of the body. Manufacturers recommend a target at 80 kV as this is where the units are calibrated.

The DRs can be calculated for different values of kV if high kV examinations are required for example chest radiography.

MCQs

1. **Which of the following contributes the most to the background dose of radiation to which the population is exposed?**
   a. Flying in a plane
   b. Radiation from nuclear discharges
   c. Medical radiation exposure
   d. Gamma radiation from buildings.

2. **The SI unit of absorbed dose is the:**
   a. Milligray
   b. Gray
   c. Sievert
   d. MilliSievert.

3. **A device which may be used to measure the X-radiation delivered to a patient is called:**
   a. Densitometer
   b. Geiger-Muller tube
   c. Photocathode
   d. Diamentor.

4. **The SI unit of dose equivalent is the:**
   a. Milligray
   b. Gray
   c. Sievert
   d. MilliSievert.

5. **An atom which loses an electron:**
   a. Is called an ion
   b. Changes its position in the periodic table
   c. Becomes negatively charged
   d. Becomes radioactive.

6. **One Gray is the absorption of:**
   a. 1 calorie of energy per kilogram of matter
   b. 1 joule of energy per kilogram of matter
   c. 1 joule per gram of matter
   d. 1 calorie per gram of matter.

7. **The equivalent dose is calculated by:**
   a. Multiplying the absorbed dose by a weighting factor which takes account of the type of radiation being used
   b. Multiplying the equivalent dose by a weighting factor which takes account of the type of radiation being used
   c. Multiplying the equivalent dose by a weighting factor which takes account of the radiosensitivity of the tissues being irradiated
   d. Multiplying the radiation exposure by a weighting factor which takes account of the radiosensitivity of the tissues being irradiated.

8. The quality factor for X-rays is:
   a. 10
   b. 20
   c. 1
   d. 100.

9. Approximately how many ionisation events will be released by a 70 keV beam:
   a. 21
   b. 210
   c. 2100
   d. 21 000

10. Which of the following is not an exposure indicator?
    a. Exposure index
    b. Sensitivity number
    c. Log median value
    d. Exposure mean.

CHAPTER 9
IMAGE DISPLAY AND MANIPULATION IN MEDICAL IMAGING

INTRODUCTION

This aim of this chapter is to explore digital imaging display and manipulation in medical imaging. All the raw data from digital medical images is manipulated by the computer before the practitioner can view them. The chapter explores the various stages in the image production pathway from the formation of the raw data matrix through to the final displayed image matrix. The computer will display an image following certain processes in a format which has been optimized either by the processes themselves or preferences determined by a practitioner. You therefore need to understand and explain relevant processes and the terminology used in the department, how a digital image is displayed on the monitor and how the image can be manipulated to enhance the quality. It finally gives a brief introduction into relevant terms and standards that are widely used within imaging departments associated with storage and transmission of images and data.

Learning objectives

The student should be able to:

- Explain terms associated with image display and manipulation, such as data matrix, spatial and contrast resolution, image interpolation filter algorithms.
- Understand and explain the principles of image manipulation, enhancement and optimization and how the operator can modify image quality.

IMAGE PRODUCTION PATHWAY

All digital images are recorded in the form of a grid known as the 'raw data image matrix'. This grid of raw data is then used to form the pixels of the displayed or reconstructed image matrix.

A great deal happens to the raw data before an image is actually displayed. **Figure 9.1** lists the main stages involved.

Raw data image matrix

This is the grid of fixed actual values collected by the computed radiography (CR)/digital radiography (DR) detector plate following exposure. Consider a chest X-ray recorded with film screen technology which has a resolution of 10 line pairs per millimetre. We have already shown how this would equate to 20 pixels per millimetre if it were a digital system. A standard chest x-ray film screen combination enclosed in a cassette of 43 × 35 cm therefore has the equivalent of a matrix of 8600 × 7000 pixels, a total of 60 200 000 pixels (or 60 mega pixels). In Chapter 6, we also discussed that spatial resolution was not the only parameter involved in image quality and that digital systems whether they are CR or DR based generally have much greater contrast resolution.

For general non-specialised radiographs, it is currently accepted that a digital system with a resolution of 10 pixels/mm^2 (equivalent to 5 lp/mm) will give similar overall image quality to film screen technology, having double the spatial resolution. A digital system would

Raw data matrix is produced
↓
Image interpolation applied
↓
Manufacturer applied system filter algorithms
↓
Manufacturer algorithms applied as part of pre-set protocols
↓
Operator/user-defined manipulation tools (LGT)
↓
Reconstructed/displayed image

(a)

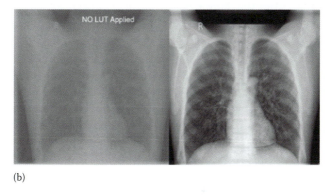

NO LUT Applied

(b)

Figure 9.1 (a) Stages involved in image manipulation; (b) raw data and processed image.

therefore require a smaller matrix of 4300 × 3500 pixels, a total of 15 050 000 (or 15 mega pixels) to offer arguably similar overall image quality.

Every pixel in the raw data matrix will have its own data value based on the incident radiation that interacted with it, effectively meaning the raw data contain a grid reference and signal value for all 15 050 000 pixels.

Display of reconstructed image matrix

The raw matrix is used to form the display image matrix. If all detail is to be displayed on the monitor, then the reconstructed image matrix has to have at least as many pixels as the original raw data matrix.

It is also important that a monitor used for image interpretation is able to display the full resolution of the raw data matrix and as such there are typically at least 4300 × 3500 pixel displays.

Lower resolution monitors are usually employed to check the technical quality in the viewing areas of most imaging departments. These are typically what is known as a 2K monitor (2048 × 2048 pixels).

Image quality and matrix size

There is a considerable effect on resolution by altering matrix size. If we increase/double the pixels in both directions from say 4 × 4 to 8 × 8, we actually have four times as many pixels. The more we increase the matrix, the better the representation of the original object.

If we consider a random shape which may represent a small body structure, we can see the effect of matrix size and how it will be recorded or displayed (**Figure 9.2**).

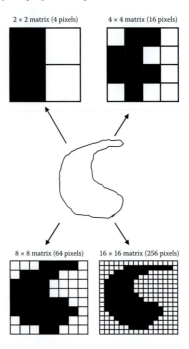

Figure 9.2 The effect of the matrix size on image display.

Although we can clearly see an improvement in how well the larger matrix represents the original object, we have to be aware that every doubling of matrix size, quadruples the number of data areas forming the matrix, which also means we require greater computer power for subsequent image manipulation and greater archive storage requirements as we have four times the data.

IMAGE INTERPOLATION

Many different types of interpolation are used simultaneously in all digital imaging modalities, e.g. linear exponential interpolation.

All interpolation algorithms fill in the gaps in the data. They are basically a mathematical filter that alters the value of data either before or after the data have been processed.

No matter how expensive, all digital systems will have minor manufacturing faults. A thin film transistor (TFT) used in a DR system, for example, will contain a few dead detector elements.

Consider a small area of a TFT-based DR system that contains a dead detector element. As this particular detector element (del) is dead, it will not send a signal so the system puts in an interpolated (educated guess) value of what it might have been. It does this by taking into account what the surrounding live dels have recorded.

IMAGE MANIPULATION

There are many ways to manipulate images, but essentially all techniques alter either the values of the pixels in the raw data matrix or reconstructed data matrix.

Before displaying the stored image data from the system memory, the data values at each address can be processed and manipulated to improve perceived image quality.

Manufacturer-defined manipulation tools

Manufacturers will incorporate some form of data manipulation which may be applied immediately to the raw data in order to maximise system efficiency and reduce noise in the system. The operator does not usually have any control over this process. These manufacturer-based algorithms are applied to the raw data matrix to improve image quality. However, their effectiveness depends on how good the original mathematics and mathematical formulae are, which is itself dependent on the accuracy of the original mathematics.

A manufacturer may also incorporate some manipulation techniques as part of pre-set anatomical protocols. A CR or DR system programmed for a chest X-ray will have a different filter algorithm applied to that of an abdominal X-ray to take account of the very different subject contrast. These filters are applied to make the most of the data collected for particular body areas and are generally very effective. There is a small caveat in that they are generally based on typical patient models and may not be as quite effective with atypical patients.

Operator-defined manipulation tools

Finally, the operator will be able to apply various manipulation techniques. The user applies these techniques if they think the original image can be improved in terms of subjective choice. They can be and are often part of a pre-set protocol and based usually on a typical patient model. These processes are operator-dependent and may not be seen as an improvement by all viewers.

Automatic or pre-programmed image reconstruction processes include:

- Windowing
- Zooming and enlarging
- Noise reduction by background subtraction
- Noise reduction by 'low-pass spatial filtering'
- Edge enhancement by 'high-pass spatial filtering'.

Windowing

Every del of the raw data matrix has its own value following exposure. Potentially, we could allocate a shade of grey on the display matrix that is directly related to the amount of radiation collected by the individual dels. However, the human eye is only really able to distinguish around 32 shades of grey on an image. Hence, we choose which signal values we wish to display by selecting a range of signal values for each shade of grey. This is a process called 'windowing'.

The window width can be increased to include a greater range of tissue types, but it also means there is less difference between various displayed tissue densities. On the other hand, window width can be narrowed to a particular tissue type, for example soft tissue, but this may mean more dense and less dense tissues, such as bone or cystic areas, may be outside the range displayed.

Zooming and enlarging

Three types are commonly available:
1. Interpolated zoom (IZ)
2. Reconstructed zoom (RZ)
3. Geometric zoom (GZ).

Manufacturers use a variety of terms and technical jargons in the literature they produce, but all the techniques will be based around the methods listed here.

Interpolated zoom

Interpolated zoom is undertaken on a workstation and involves manipulation of the raw data matrix. Interpolation algorithms of one sort or another are used under a variety of manufacturers' trade names to produce a zoomed image.

The raw data pixels are enlarged to produce a bigger image by simple magnification. However, the pixels in the new image are now much larger, so a second process is applied by dividing the larger 'real' pixels into smaller but interpolated pixels. The result looks reasonable as pixel size is reduced relative to image enlargement, therefore potentially increasing spatial resolution (SR).

However, the data values of the new smaller tissue volumes tend to be an average of the original larger tissue volume. So while pixels represent smaller volumes they do not represent true patient data, but rather arithmetic averages (interpolations).

Reconstructed zoom

Reconstructed zoom is undertaken on a workstation and involves manipulation of the raw data matrix. It allows reconstruction of smaller areas and uses the original data set.

It is very effective if the raw data matrix is smaller than the display matrix size, as we effectively have more information to reconstruct than is actually being used. However, once the display matrix is greater than the raw data matrix, it effectively requires interpolation and is no longer true image zooming. As such it may or may not use zooming interpolation algorithms, dependent on original data sampling and data set size in relation to display matrix.

Geometric zoom

True geometric zoom requires the movement of the detector plate and tube relative to the object, thereby altering the geometry (**Figure 9.3**). It means that a small object is projected over many more dels with greater coverage of the detector plate, in comparison with the other two techniques. This technique is more commonly known as 'macroradiography'.

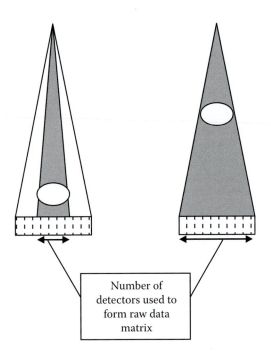

Figure 9.3 Geometric zoom.

NOISE REDUCTION BY BACKGROUND SUBTRACTION

In its simplest form, the signal values are all reduced by the same amount, reducing not only the level of noise, but also the useable signal. As such the raw signal-to-noise ratio is actually very similar.

If we consider a data set of 16 pixels, the height of the bars represents the actual signal collected by the relevant del of the imaging system. All dels give off a small amount of noise with any real signal being added to this background noise (**Figure 9.4**).

If these values were displayed, the image would look something like the grid of pixels shown in **Figure 9.5**, with the low signal values in pixels 1, 2, 10 and 16 being just above background noise.

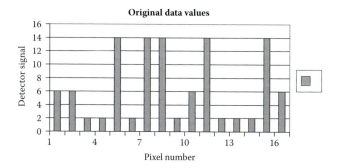

Figure 9.4 Actual signal values (raw data).

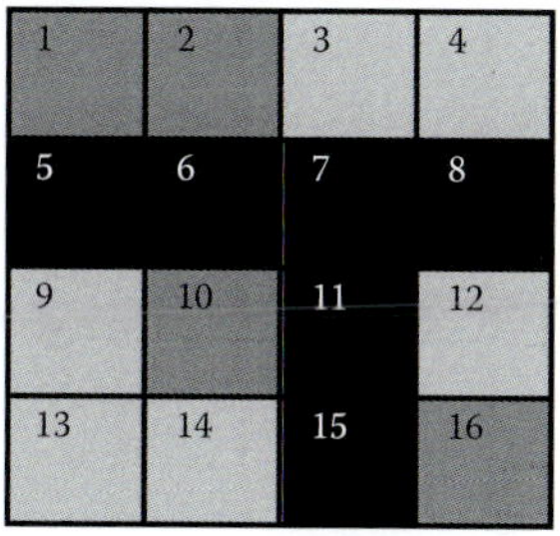

Figure 9.5 How this raw data might reconstruct.

If we apply background subtraction, all pixels are reduced equally, reducing the background noise of the system. However, it also reduces the signal values by the same amount (**Figure 9.6**).

It is then possible to subjectively restore contrast by increasing signal values by appropriate contrast enhancement or windowing (**Figure 9.7**).

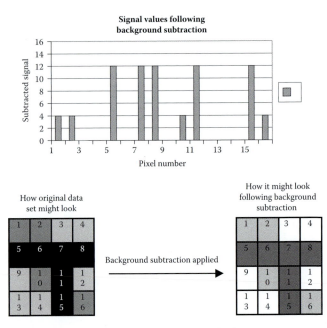

Figure 9.6 New signal values following background subtraction.

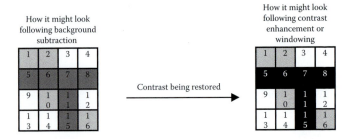

Figure 9.7 Illustrates the effect on the pixels when background subtraction and contrast enhancement algorithms are applied.

NOISE REDUCTION BY 'LOW-PASS SPATIAL FILTERING'

This is a form of 'image smoothing'.

We need to consider the pixels making up the image matrix in groups of nine pixels. The grey scale value of the central pixel of this group of nine (as indicated by C in **Figure 9.8**) is added as a proportion of the average value of the eight surrounding pixels (S in **Figure 9.8**).

This proportion of the average value can be changed depending on how much we want to smooth the image. This essentially leads to very small areas of light or dark being removed from the data, whether they are noise or real data. The small detector values relating to pixels 1, 2, 10 and 16 could be smoothed out of the data if this technique is applied too aggressively (**Figure 9.9**).

It is effective at reducing noise, but also results in a slight reduction in spatial and contrast resolution.

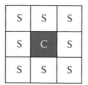

Figure 9.8 Shows a central pixel surrounded by 8 pixels used in this process.

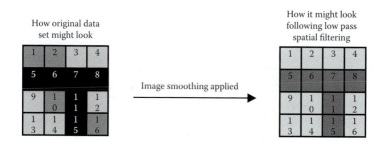

How original data set might look

Image smoothing applied

How it might look following low pass spatial filtering

Figure 9.9 Effect of image smoothing.

No edge enhancement | With edge enhancement

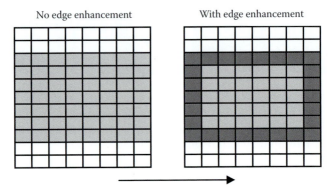

Figure 9.10 Edge enhancement.

EDGE ENHANCEMENT BY 'HIGH-PASS SPATIAL FILTERING'

This technique examines the data set and detects where the data change from a high attenuating area to a low attenuating area. The pixels nearest to the edge of this change are given an artificially high signal value effectively outlining the structure (**Figure. 9.10**).

STANDARDS

Traditionally, no or very few common standards were available for different pieces of equipment by different manufacturers. With modern equipment, it is important that an image produced by a particular equipment manufacturer might need to be manipulated, displayed and stored on a piece of equipment by a different manufacturer.

A common standard was produced to allow this to happen and is known as 'digital imaging and communications in medicine' (DICOM).

DICOM information contains a number of elements including information such as patient details and obviously the post-manipulated images themselves (as pixel values). A fully DICOM-compatible data set will contain additional information, such as the imaging protocols used, raw data values, as well as details of any manipulation filters already applied which are important for future manipulation of the image.

In addition to DICOM, there are a number of other standards enabling picture archive and communications systems (PACS), as well as wider teleradiology systems, to operate. Although slightly beyond the remit of this book, some of these standards warrant a mention and include:

1. IEEE 802.3 (ethernet). This stems from computer networks and is associated with the physical layer on which the image data passes (network plugs, sockets, wires, switches and network cards).
2. IEEE 802.5 (token ring). Similar to ethernet standard, except that a 'token' is required to gain access to image data. A good example might be a dongle, which is a small device similar to a USB memory stick that has to be physically plugged into a computer in order to access certain images and data.
3. TCP/IP (transmission control protocol/internet protocol). This is a standard to ensure that data are transmitted over the internet without image or data degradation or corruption.
4. HL-7 (Health Level 7) is basically to ensure that a radiology information system (RIS) can talk to PACS and the hospital information system (HIS) systems. It also enables one hospital PACS, RIS and HIS to talk to another hospital's set-up.

MCQs

1. **A digital system with a resolution of 10 pixels/mm^2 is:**
   a. Equivalent to 10 lp/mm
   b. Equivalent to 20 lp/mm
   c. Equivalent to 15 lp/mm
   d. Equivalent to 5 lp/mm.
2. **If we double the image matrix size from 256×256 to 512×512, the data are:**
   a. Twice the resolution
   b. Twice the resolution, but four times the data
   c. Four times the data and four times the resolution
   d. Four times the data, but half the resolution.

3. **A 2K monitor will have approximately:**
   a. 2000 pixels
   b. 4000 pixels
   c. 40 000 pixels
   d. 4 000 000 pixels.

4. **A full resolution monitor needs to display at least**
   a. 3500 × 3500 pixels
   b. 4300 × 3500 pixels
   c. 4300 × 4300 pixels
   d. 2000 × 2000 pixels.

5. **The human eye is only really able to distinguish around:**
   a. 60 shades of grey on an image
   b. 10 shades of grey on an image
   c. 4000 shades of grey on an image
   d. 32 shades of grey on an image.

6. **Windowing:**
   a. Allows images to be altered in size to fit the display
   b. Changes the contrast and brightness of the image
   c. Allows certain tissue densities to be divided into 32 discrete shades of grey for display
   d. Can be used to increase the number of pixels displayed.

7. **Interpolated zoom:**
   a. Requires the movement of the detector plate and tube relative to the object
   b. Is true image zooming
   c. Is a two-stage process that simply enlarges the pixels and then subdivides them to produce new smaller pixels
   d. Is an artificial image zoom.

8. **Macro-radiography is another name for:**
   a. Geometric zoom
   b. Interpolated zoom
   c. Reconstructed zoom
   d. Magnification.

9. **Noise reduction by background subtraction:**
   a. Is where the signal values are all reduced by the same amount
   b. Takes account of the average of the surrounding pixels
   c. Increases contrast and spatial resolution
   d. Decreases contrast and special resolution.

10. **A common standard for transferring data files between manu-facturers is:**
    a. SITCOM
    b. DIDCOM
    c. DICOM
    d. OFCOM

CHAPTER 10
RADIATION PROTECTION AND SAFETY

INTRODUCTION

The aim of this chapter is to give the practitioner an understanding of the basic principles of radiation protection and safety. It is essential that any practitioner operating within an imaging department and using ionising radiation has a sound basis for their knowledge. You need to comprehend and be able to explain the factors affecting the protection of staff, patients and the general public.

The primary purpose of radiation protection when using medical radiation is to reduce the associated risks to staff, patients and visitors to the imaging department to a minimal acceptable level. It should be remembered that the majority of anyone's radiation dose will originate from naturally occurring radiations and there is little or nothing that can be done to reduce that dose. However, man-made radiation constitutes approximately 14 per cent of an individual's total radiation dose, 85–90 per cent of which (i.e. 12 per cent of the total radiation dose) arises from the use of ionising radiation in medical and dental practice and here you can have an influence.

The purpose of diagnostic imaging is to produce images of diagnostic quality at the lowest radiation dose. Therefore, the ultimate consideration is to provide a diagnostic image and manage the patient effectively as a result of the test.

LEGISLATION

There are two main pieces of legislation in Europe which determine protection of staff, patients and the general public. These are:
1. Ionising Radiations Regulation (IRR'99)
2. The Ionising Radiation (Medical Exposure) Regulations 2000 (IR(ME)R 2000)

IRR'99

The protection of staff is largely controlled through the application of IRR'99. The legislation makes stringent requirements of employers to protect not only their staff, but also patients and members of the general public (a category which includes everyone who might be found in a hospital who could not be classified as either a patient or an employee). This document, among many other things establishes:
- Designation of classified persons. Defined as those employees who are likely to receive an effective dose in excess of 6 mSv per year or an equivalent dose which is likely to exceed three-tenths of any relevant dose limit.
- Notification and investigation of overexposure.
- Dose-equivalent limits for radiation workers and it is the enforcement of such limits that have eliminated the illnesses and premature deaths seen in early radiation workers who were exposed to very large doses of ionising radiation, largely through ignorance.
- The application of the dose equivalent limits for different categories of workers and also the ALARP principle for

the protection of non-employees. ALARP means as low as reasonably practicable (social and economic factors being taken into consideration) and refers to the radiation doses administered by the workers/employees.

Applying the ALARP principle is one of your main considerations when undertaking an X-ray. This must be applied not only to the patient but to visitors, other staff and, of course, yourself. Largely this is done by ensuring the justificative process and ensuring that all X-ray room doors are closed. All non-essential staff are excluded during X-ray examinations.

IR(ME)R 2000

These regulations are intended to protect individuals against the dangers of ionising radiation while undergoing medical exposures. These include diagnostic procedures such as X-rays, computed tomography (CT) scans and nuclear medicine examinations, as well as treatment such as radiotherapy, irrespective of where they are undertaken, e.g. hospital department, dental practice, chiropractic clinic. Medical exposures undertaken for research purposes are also covered by these regulations.

The regulations define the duty-holders who carry responsibility under IR(ME)R 2000. These are:

- The employer who is (normally the NHS Trust in the hospital-based environment) is the body responsible for putting all the necessary procedures and protocols in place to ensure that the IR(ME)R 2000 regulations can be fully applied
- The referrer, a registered health care professional (e.g. a medical or dental practitioner, radiographer, chiropodist, etc.) who is entitled, in accordance with the employer's procedures, to refer patients for medical exposures
- The practitioner, a registered health care professional who is entitled in accordance with the employer's procedures and whose primary responsibility is justification of the individual medical exposure (e.g. the radiographer or radiologist)
- The operator, a person who is entitled in accordance with the employer's procedures to undertake the medical exposure (e.g. an assistant practitioner or a student radiographer).

Some of the main points to arise from the implementation of IR(ME)R 2000 are:

- Justification
    - No person shall carry out a medical exposure unless it has been justified by the referrer or practitioner as showing a net benefit to the individual.
    - It has been authorised by the practitioner or, where paragraph (5) applies, the operator.
- Diagnostic reference levels (DRL)
    - The employer must set DRLs and provide guidance and procedures on how they are to be used. A diagnostic reference level is set for each standard radiological investigation. They should also be set for interventional procedures, nuclear medicine investigations and radiotherapy planning procedures.

Optimisation

- The practitioner and the operator, to the extent of their respective involvement in a medical exposure, shall ensure that doses arising from the exposure are kept as low as reasonably practicable consistent with the intended purpose, of the exposure.
- The operator shall select equipment and methods to ensure that for each medical exposure, the dose of ionising radiation to the individual undergoing the exposure is as low as reasonably practicable and consistent with the intended diagnostic or therapeutic purpose and in doing so shall pay special attention to:
    - Careful/precise technique to minimise repeat examinations
    - Quality assurance of equipment.
    - Optimisation of exposure factors to provide a diagnostic image within the DRLs set for each procedure.
- Clinical audit of procedures and exposures.

Training

- No practitioner or operator shall carry out a medical exposure without having been adequately trained.

The inspectorate of the Health and Safety Executive has responsibility for the enforcement of each of the above regulations.

It is impossible in a pocket-book such as this to provide a full coverage of all of the ionising radiation regulations. It is therefore recommended that you use published guidance, such as appropriate legislative information on government links.

Local rules and systems of work

Drawn up in accordance with Regulation 17 of the Ionising Radiations Regulations 1999 (IRR'99). They state all users must read them and sign a statement that they have read them, understood them and will comply with the local rules. There are certain responsibilities under the act, as outlined below.

Responsibilities

- Employer
    - Compliance with regulations
    - Appointment of radiation protection advisor (RPA)
- All employees
    - Ensure their own and colleagues' safety
    - Use relevant protection devices

There must also be designated areas:

- X-ray room is a controlled area.
- Warning signs must be present and lit when an exposure is taking place.
- Entry/exit doors must be closed during exposure and staff must not enter.

Radiation protection of staff

Staff must ensure they are not accidentally exposed to radiation and have a legal requirement to protect themselves from risk. This can be achieved in a number of ways:

- X-ray and gamma camera rooms are designed to minimise the dose to staff.
- Only staff necessary should be present when an exposure is made.
- Shielding
    - Stand behind protective screen when an exposure is made.

- Wear personal protective equipment (PPE) when undertaking fluoroscopy or exposures with mobile equipment.
- Radioactive sources must be shielded.
- Distance
  - Use the inverse square law to stand far enough away from the X-ray or radiation source. There is a 2 m controlled area from the image intensifier in which the staff must wear appropriate PPE.
- Time
- Staff should minimise the amount of time spent in fluoroscopy or close to a radioactive source.

Staff may also be monitored to ensure they do not exceed the legal dose limits for workers.

DOSE LIMITS

- Adult employees 20 mSv per calender year.
- Trainees under 18 years, 6 mSv
- Others, 1 mSv
- Comforters and carers (five years), 5 mSv
- Dose to fetus for the remainer of the pregnancy, 1 mSv
- Dose to abdomen of woman of reproductive capacity in three-month period, 1.3 mSv.

PHYSICAL, CHEMICAL AND BIOLOGICAL EFFECTS OF IONISING RADIATION

We now know that as X- and gamma rays penetrate matter they have the ability to ionise it (which is why we call them 'ionising radiations'). When energy is absorbed from the radiation by matter, it has the ability to split electrons from their associated atoms or molecules, leading to the production of a negative ion (the dissociated electron) and a positive ion (the remainder of the atom or molecule, now minus one of its negatively charged electrons).

This initial process can subsequently give rise to a four-stage process:

- Stage 1. Energy from the photon of radiation is absorbed by atoms or molecules of the material giving rise to the physical process of ionisation.
- Stage 2. The electron(s) ejected from the atom(s) may have sufficient energy to ionise other atoms in which case secondary ionisation has occurred and highly reactive free radicals are produced.
- Stage 3. The free radicals can then go on to interact with other cellular chemicals to produce chemical changes.
- Stage 4. The chemical changes can cause the cell function to change, which is itself a biological change within tissue.

The biological effects of ionising radiation can be grouped under two headings:

CANCER EFFECTS

The likelihood of this effect occurring is governed by the laws of probability and the chance of it occurring is therefore directly related to the dose of ionising radiation received. The guiding principles arising from this probability-related effect are two fold:

1. There is no 'threshold' limit below which a stochastic effect cannot occur. However, the greater the dose received, the greater the risk of the effect occurring. It therefore follows that if we calculate dose equivalent limits for the radiations at our disposal, we can use them to calculate the statistical risk that an individual runs by exceeding that limit.
2. While the chance of a cancer effect occurring may be probability-related, the severity of any resultant effect will not be. We know from statistical records that populations which are exposed to ionising radiations (over and above natural background radiation which everyone receives to a lesser or greater extent, depending largely on where they live) have a greater risk of developing cancer. However, if the disease is contracted, its severity will not be related to the radiation dose received.

There is a much reduced risk of developing a cancer following a low-dose chest X-ray than there would be following a high-dose examination, such as a CT scan of the chest. However, if a cancer did result from either examination, its rate and extent of progression would be related to the genetic make up of the individual, not the dose of radiation which may have caused it.

There are two types of cancer effects resulting from exposure to ionising radiations:

Somatic effects

The main one being cancer itself. The risk of developing a cancer from a medical irradiation is related to the dose of radiation received as we have said previously. However, the general risk is very small across all examinations. It is clear from research data that some tissues are more sensitive and therefore at greater risk of developing a malignancy than others. This can be helpful in that most cancer cells develop more quickly than their surrounding tissues and therefore may respond to the use of ionising radiation as a treatment to destroy or shrink the tumour.

The downside though is that some naturally occurring tissues, such as stem cells and fetal cells develop extremely rapidly and are therefore at greater risk also. It is for this reason that we have radiation protection regulations which protect vulnerable groups such as pregnant women and those who think they may be pregnant (see Special protection measures for women of reproductive capacity), and we aim to minimise the risk of cancer development to all by applying the ALARP principle every time we undertake an X-ray examination.

Hereditary (genetic) effects

These are effects which are caused by radiation-induced damage to the genetic material carried in an individual's germ cells carried in the ova or spermatozoa. Ionising radiation can cause biological damage to genes which may cause faulty combinations of chromosomes to occur. Such damage can only show itself in future generations and may or may not become part of the broader human gene pool depending on whether the resulting individuals themselves, go on to reproduce.

The aim in any case is to make every effort to reduce the radiation dose received to the gonads to an absolute minimum – using sound radiographic techniques and appropriate protective devices – as the effects are unpredictable and potentially far-reaching.

Heritable (also known as deterministic) effects are defined by two properties

1. Their severity will increase with increasing dose (i.e. the effect is proportional to the dose).
2. There is usually a threshold below which the effect will not occur.

It is reasonable to say that heritable effects will always occur if a threshold dose is achieved (unlike stochastic effects which may occur whatever the dose received). Deterministic effects are associated with what we would consider to be in diagnostic imaging terms, very large radiation doses of an order of magnitude only experienced as a result of nuclear or other radiation-related accidents. They may occur in radiotherapy.

Examples of deterministic effects might be:

- Radiation burns (also called 'erythema' or skin reddening)
- Radiation-induced cataracts and sterility.

Erythema will occur from 1 to 24 hours after a radiation dose of 2 Sieverts and cataracts will occur after 2–10 Sieverts have been received, but may take many years to develop. To apply some perspective for diagnostic radiographers, 1 Sievert is equivalent to around 50 000 chest X-rays or 100 whole-body CT scans.

In very basic terms, the aim of the radiographer when undertaking a radiographic investigation is, first and foremost, to secure an optimum diagnostic image while at the same time, minimising the risk of a cancer event and subjecting the patient to no risk at all of a heritable event occurring.

SPECIAL PROTECTION MEASURES FOR WOMEN OF REPRODUCTIVE CAPACITY

The fetus, as has been mentioned previously, is a structure which is relatively sensitive to ionising radiation, largely due to the rate of cellular reproduction. The term 'relative' in this context compares the fetus to a fully grown individual.

There are many different interpretations of how the potentially pregnant or pregnant woman (and therefore, by definition, the fetus) should be considered when they are referred for an X-ray examination and it is essential that those newly appointed to a Trust's team of radiographers ensure that they aware of the local interpretation of the guidelines and recommendations.

The 1984 International Commission for Radiation Protection (ICRP) guideline which is still in use today states that:

> During the first 10 days following the onset of a menstrual period, there can be no risk of pregnancy since no conception will have occurred. The risk to a child who had previously been irradiated *in utero* during the remainder of the 4 week period following the onset of menstruation is likely to be so small that there need be no special limitation on exposures required within these 4 weeks.

This superseded the previous ICRP recommendation of 1970 which stated that:

> Women of reproductive capacity should only be X-rayed within 10 days of the commencement of their last menstrual period.

The 1970 recommendation, for what are probably obvious reasons, came to be known as the '10-day rule' and consequently, the 1984 recommendation was referred to as the '28-day rule'.

Each of these 'rules' quite often finds a place in departmental protocols; the 10-day rule, because of its more stringent implications, tends to find favour when higher-dose examinations are undertaken, such as barium enemas or CT scans of the abdominopelvic region, but is often seen as too restrictive from a clinical perspective to be applied to plain X-ray examinations. The so-called 28-day rule is normally applied for routine X-ray examinations of any anatomical area between the diaphragm and the knees of women of child-bearing age.

Determining 'child-bearing age' can however, pose a dilemma in itself, but this is usually overcome by the setting of an age range when the appropriate questions must be asked prior to the X-ray examination.

In many cases, that age-range is between 12 and 55 years, but you must check local protocols prior to commencing employment in a particular place as this is a very variable parameter.

In addition to the 1984 recommendation above, the National Radiological Protection Board (NRPB) also issued supporting guidelines which will stand you well in the practice environment if you commit them to memory:

- Any woman who has an overdue or missed period should be treated as though she were pregnant;
- If the woman cannot answer 'No' to the question: 'Are you or might you be pregnant?', then she should be regarded as if she were pregnant.

If the clinical indications are that an exposure should be made where the primary beam will irradiate the fetus, then great care must be taken to minimise the number of exposures and the absorbed dose per exposure, but without compromising the diagnostic value of the investigation.

Provided good collimation and properly shielded equipment is used, radiographs remote from the fetus may be done safely at any time during the pregnancy.

REPORTING OF RADIATION INCIDENTS

An overexposure may be defined as an exposure in excess of a relevant dose limit (employee or member of the public). This is an exposure much greater than intended, therefore is a dose to a patient that exceeds the guideline multiplying factors in Health and Safety Executive (HSE) publication PM77.

The notification guidelines are broadly representative of patient exposure, i.e. effective dose or mean glandular dose. Suitable measurements for determining these quantities are:

- Dose–area product (DAP) metre
- Duration of exposure
- Product of tube current and time (mAs)
- Volume of tissue irradiated
- Activity administered.

Radiographers undertaking X-rays of extremities, skull, dentition and chest must notify the HSE if the dose is 20 times more than intended.

MCQs

1. **Deterministic effects of radiation include:**
   a. Cataracts
   b. Sterility
   c. Erythema
   d. Leukaemia.

2. **Stochastic effects of radiation include:**
   a. Carcinogenesis
   b. Heridity
   c. Erythema
   d. Leukaemia

3. **Manmade radiations account for what percentage of background dose:**
   a. 3%
   b. 10%
   c. 14%
   d. 20%.

4. **The person responsible for justification of an exposure to X-rays is the:**
   a. The employer
   b. The operator
   c. The practitioner
   d. The referrer.

5. **The operator is responsible for:**
   a. Setting DRL's for each examination
   b. Writing the local rules
   c. Optimising the radiation dose to the patient for each examination (ALARA)
   d. Training referrers to fill in the request form correctly.

6. **The controlled area extends to which distance from the X-ray source (tube)**
   a. 1 metres
   b. 2 metres
   c. 3 metres
   d. 4 metres.

7. Designated workers are defined as those employees who are likely to receive:
   a. 20 mSv per year
   b. 1 mSv per year
   c. 5 mSv per year
   d. 6 mSv per year.

8. **Cancer effect of ionising radiation have the following characteristics:**
   a. No threshold dose below which it cannot occur
   b. A threshold dose below which it cannot occur
   c. The same risk regardless of the radiation dose
   d. The effect is proportional to the dose.

9. **At what point should overexposure for radiography be notified to the HSE?**
   a. Twice the intended exposure
   b. Four times the intended exposure
   c. 10 x the intended exposure
   d. 20 x the intended exposure.

10. **What is the aim of the X-ray examination?**
   a. Optimum images with no risk
   b. Optimum images with minimum risk
   c. Optimum images regardless of the radiation dose
   d. Optimum images with risk of heritable effects.

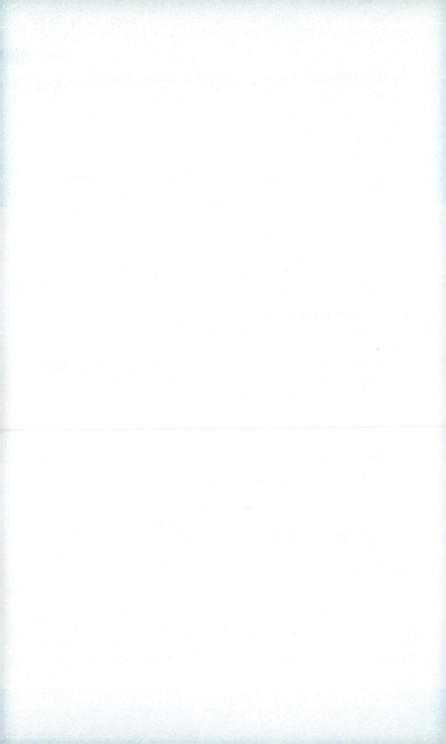

CHAPTER 11
RISK–BENEFIT

INTRODUCTION

The aim of this chapter is to give the practitioner an understanding of the basic principles of risk–benefit. It is essential that any practitioner using ionising radiation has the knowledge and skills to enter a dialogue into with patients concerning risk–benefit. You need to comprehend and be able to explain the benefits of examinations using X-rays and the factors affecting radiation dose

> **Learning objectives**
>
> The student should be able to:
> - Understand and explain the basic principles of risk–benefit.
> - Have a dialogue with patients and staff on the risk–benefit of examinations using X- and gamma-radiations.

RISK–BENEFIT ANALYSIS

Risk–benefit analysis is one of the best tools for managing risk on a daily basis in all walks of life (you probably use it for yourself dozens of times a day), but its value as a key weapon in the armoury of the radiographer has to be considered differently as you will be utilizing it in your professional capacity on a daily basis, not for your own benefit, but for that of others.

While risk–benefit analysis can, at least in theory, be applied for every patient examination we undertake, the same cannot be said when we consider the radiation dose that workers such as radiographers and other health professionals receive. There is no benefit for these people from the dose of radiation they could potentially receive (if you discount earning an income for now) and therefore radiation protection has to be considered differently for this group of people. Risk analysis is still a very big part of the process of protecting radiation workers but in this case, has to be considered as a non-beneficial risk.

We now have a clear understanding that the use of X-rays carries with it, on the one hand, associated dangers or risks, yet on the other, distinct benefits for mankind (can you imagine a twenty-first century hospital providing its services without using X-rays or radio-isotopes for that matter in either a diagnostic or therapeutic capacity?). It therefore follows that it is necessary to control some of the factors associated with the use of X-rays. Radiation legislation in the UK requires that no one should be irradiated intentionally unless there is a valid clinical indication. In making this judgement, the clinician must determine that the benefit to the patient in having the examination will outweigh the risk. This is the process of justification and if the result of having the X-ray examination will change the clinical management of the patient then that examination can be said to be justified.

You do have to be aware, however, that requesting an X-ray to exclude an injury or a disease process can be perfectly justifiable also, providing it is not possible to be reasonably sure of the outcome by other, less risky means. An example of 'less risky' in this case might be a thorough clinical examination.

So justification is the first step in a radiation protection strategy because the best way to reduce the radiation dose to the patient is not to undertake the examination in the first place, if this is considered to be an appropriate course of action. The justification of an X-ray examination is a two-stage process and should be the responsibility of both the requesting clinician along with the radiographer responsible for undertaking the request. Determining whether an examination is justified will vary depending on factors such as the age of the individual, the pregnancy status or the availability of other diagnostic procedures.

BENEFITS OF X-RAY EXAMINATIONS

The benefits of having X-ray procedures are associated with managing the treatment and/or diagnosis of the patient. These may include:

- Saving the person's life by providing the correct diagnosis which may not be able to be made without the use of X-rays, e.g. chest X-ray to demonstrate extent of pathology.
- Giving the patient the correct treatment as a result of the correct diagnosis.
- Eliminating disease/disorders which affect the management of the patient, e.g. determining if a patient has a fracture and how best to manage the patient's fracture.
- Managing the treatment of a patient by imaging the response to treatment, e.g. images to determine the effect of radiotherapy.
- Making a diagnosis with an examination which has less morbidity and mortality than an alternative test, e.g. computed tomography (CT), rather than invasive surgery.

RISKS FROM X- AND γ-RADIATION

There is no safe dose limit and all doses carry some risk. The purpose of a risk–benefit discussion should therefore justify the examination to the patient, discuss the need for the examination and quantify the risk. The Health Protection Agency produces an excellent leaflet, called 'X-ray Safety Leaflet' which outlines the common imaging procedures and levels of risk for common X-ray and isotope procedures. To quote them,

> You will be glad to know that the radiation doses used for X-ray examinations or isotope scans are many thousands of times too low to produce immediate harmful effects, such as skin burns or radiation sickness. The only effect on the patient that is known to be possible at these low doses is a very slight increase in the chance of cancer occurring many years or even decades after the exposure.

It also gives approximate estimates of the chance or risk that a particular examination or scan might result in a radiation-induced cancer later in the lifetime of the patient.

There are a number of ways of describing the risk. These include:

- Equivalent background dose, expressed in equivalent period of natural background radiation, e.g. a few days to several years.
- Statistical risk, expressed in numbers, e.g. risk of cancer is 1 in 1 000 000.
- Comparisons to general risks of cancer, i.e. the population have a 1 in 3 chance of getting cancer.
- Comparison to everyday activities:
  - For example, airline flights are very safe with the risk of a crash being well below 1 in 1 000 000.
  - A chest X-ray exposes you to the same risk as a 4-hour flight.
  - Smoking or drinking alcohol.
  - Driving or undertaking dangerous sports, such as skydiving.
- Lost life expectancy, given in days.

The purpose of managing radiation dose in diagnostic procedures using X-ray or gamma radiation is to avoid deterministic health effects and to reduce the probability of stochastic health effects of ionising radiation. If the DNA within cell(s) is damaged there are three possible outcomes:

1. The cell(s) die. The death of a few cells in the millions within the human body has no significant effect.
2. Significant numbers are damaged to observe a clinical effect, either immediately (erythema) or delayed (cataracts).
3. The damage is incorrectly repaired leading to mutation of the DNA. These cell(s) may subsequently die or may lead to radiation-induced malignancy.

Practitioners must be educated in the risks and benefits and the radiation dose given from X-ray procedures. Whichever one you decide to use, make sure you have the correct information at hand and always discuss risk versus benefit. You can also use the principles of justification and optimisation to inform the patient that X-rays are not undertaken without a valid clinical reason. Any examinations will optimise the exposure and use the lowest dose compatible with making a diagnosis (ALARP). Don't forget the patient always has the right to decide not to have the examination.

MCQs

1. **Discussions with patients should always include:**
   a. The risks
   b. The benefits
   c. Risk-benefit
   d. Statistical analysis of the risk.

2. **Risk of X-rays include:**
   a. Saving the person's life.
   b. Giving the patient the correct treatment as a result of the correct diagnosis
   c. Making a diagnosis with an examination which has less morbidity and mortality than an alternative test
   d. Hair loss.

3. **The risk of developing a carcinoma in the general population is:**
   a. 1 in 2
   b. 1 in 3
   c. 1 in 4
   d. 1 in 5.

4. **The everyday risk associated with a chest X-ray is approximately flying for:**
   a. 1 hour
   b. 2 hours
   c. 3 hours
   d. 4 hours.

5. **An X-ray described as minimal risk is:**
   a. Less than 1 in 1,000,000
   b. 1,000,000 to 100,000
   c. 100,000 to 10,000
   d. 10,000 to 1,000.

6. **The following are ways to minimise the risk from X-rays:**
   a. Justification
   b. Optimisation
   c. DRL's
   d. All of the above.

7. **The purpose of managing radiation dose is:**
   a. To avoid deterministic effects
   b. To avoid stochastic effects
   c. To avoid deterministic effects and minimise stochastic effects
   d. To increase the probability of stochastic effects.

8. **Who is jointly responsible for justifying an exposure to X-rays?**
   a. Practitioner and referrer
   b. Referrer and employer
   c. Patient and employer
   d. Patient and referrer.

9. **Which of the following statements is true?**
   a. The patient must have an X-ray if the referrer sends them to the imaging department
   b. The patient has the right to refuse an X-ray
   c. Practitioners must X-ray patients if the referrer tells them to do it
   d. Requesting physicians have no obligation to inform the patient of the risk from an X-ray.

10. **For an X-ray to be justified it must:**
    a. Clearly demonstrate the suspected injury or pathology
    b. Have a risk of 1,000,000 to 100,000 of resulting in a radiation-induced cancer
    c. Change the management of the patient
    d. Have an exposure within the DRL.

ANSWERS TO MCQ'S

CHAPTER 1

1. c
2. d
3. a
4. c
5. c
6. d
7. d
8. c
9. c
10. d

CHAPTER 2

1. b
2. c
3. d
4. b
5. b
6. a
7. b
8. c
9. c
10. b

CHAPTER 3

1. b
2. d

3. a
4. a
5. c
6. b
7. a
8. c
9. c
10. c

CHAPTER 4

1. d
2. a
3. b
4. b
5. c
6. c
7. a
8. a
9. d
10. a

CHAPTER 5

1. b
2. c
3. d
4. a
5. c
6. a
7. c
8. b
9. a
10. d

CHAPTER 6

1. a
2. a
3. b
4. d
5. c
6. c
7. b
8. d
9. a
10. c

CHAPTER 7

1. a
2. c
3. d
4. d
5. a
6. c
7. c
8. b
9. a
10. c

CHAPTER 8

1. c
2. b
3. d
4. c
5. a
6. b

7. a
8. c
9. c
10. d

CHAPTER 9

1. b
2. b
3. d
4. b
5. d
6. c
7. c
8. a
9. a
10. c

CHAPTER 10

1. d
2. c
3. c
4. c
5. c
6. b
7. d
8. a
9. d
10. b

CHAPTER 11

1. c
2. d
3. b
4. d
5. b
6. d
7. c
8. a
9. b
10. c

CHAPTER FORMULAS

CHAPTER 1

$$\text{Magnification} = \frac{\text{FRD}}{\text{FOD}}$$

$$\text{Area of unsharpness} = \frac{\text{Focus} \times \text{ORD}}{\text{FRD} - \text{ORD}}$$

CHAPTER 2

$$\frac{\text{mAs} \times \text{kVp}^4}{\text{grid factor} \times \text{FRD}^2} = \frac{\text{mAs} \times \text{kVp}^4}{\text{grid factor} \times \text{FRD}^2}$$

$$\frac{1 \times 70^4}{2 \times 150^2} = \frac{x \times 70^4}{1 \times 180^2}$$

$$x = \frac{70^4 \times 180^2}{70^4 \times 2 \times 150^2}$$

$$\frac{10000}{100}$$

$$a = r \sin\theta.$$

$$1 \propto \frac{1}{d^2}$$

CHAPTER 3

$(mass\ number)12$
$(atomic\ number)6$ C

1 Newton = 1 kg × m/s^2

1 joule = Newton × metres

1A = 1 coulomb of charge flowing/s

$^{12}_{6}C$

$\dfrac{1}{1840}$

CHAPTER 5

$\mu = \tau + \sigma.$

$\dfrac{\mu}{\rho} = \dfrac{\tau}{\rho} + \dfrac{\sigma}{\rho}$

attenuation = absorption + scatter.

$\dfrac{\tau}{\rho} \propto Z^3$

$\dfrac{\tau}{\rho} \propto \dfrac{1}{E^3}$

$$\frac{\sigma}{\rho} \propto \frac{Z^3}{E^3}$$

$$\frac{\sigma}{\rho} \propto \frac{1}{E}$$

$$- \propto \text{electron density}$$

CHAPTER 7

$$Ug = \frac{Focal\ spot\ size \times ORD}{FRD}$$

INDEX

Index

Index